Introduction to Many-Facet Rasch Measurement

Language Testing and Evaluation

Series editors: Rüdiger Grotjahn and Günther Sigott

Volume 22

Zu Qualitätssicherung und Peer Review der vorliegenden Publikation

Die Qualität der in dieser Reihe erscheinenden Arbeiten wird vor der Publikation durch die Herausgeber der Reihe geprüft.

Notes on the quality assurance and peer review of this publication

Prior to publication, the quality of the work published in this series is reviewed by the editors of the series.

Thomas Eckes

Introduction to Many-Facet Rasch Measurement

Analyzing and Evaluating Rater-Mediated Assessments

2nd Revised and Updated Edition

PETER LANG
EDITION

Bibliographic Information published by the Deutsche Nationalbibliothek
The Deutsche Nationalbibliothek lists this publication in the Deutsche Nationalbibliografie; detailed bibliographic data is available in the internet at http://dnb.d-nb.de.

Library of Congress Cataloging-in-Publication Data
Eckes, Thomas.
Introduction to many-facet rasch measurement : analyzing and evaluating rater-mediated assessments / Thomas Eckes. — Second revised and updated edition.
pages cm
Includes bibliographical references and index.
ISBN 978-3-631-65615-0
1. Educational tests and measurements. 2. Education—Mathematical models. 3. Rasch models. I. Title.
LB3051.E235 2015
371.26—dc23

2015024536

ISSN 1612-815X
ISBN 978-3-631-65615-0 (Print)
E-ISBN 978-3-653-04844-5 (E-Book)
DOI 10.3726/978-3-653-04844-5

Peter Lang Edition is an Imprint of Peter Lang GmbH.

Peter Lang – Frankfurt am Main · Bern · Bruxelles · New York · Oxford · Warszawa · Wien

This publication has been peer reviewed.

www.peterlang.com

Contents

Preface to the First Edition

This book grew out of times of doubt and disillusionment, times when I realized that our raters, all experienced professionals specifically trained in rating the performance of examinees on writing and speaking tasks of a high-stakes language test, were unable to reach agreement in the final scores they awarded to examinees. What first seemed to be a sporadic intrusion of inevitable human error, soon turned out to follow an undeniable, clear-cut pattern: Interrater agreement and reliability statistics revealed that ratings of the very same performance differed from one another to an extent that was totally unacceptable, considering the consequences for examinees' study and life plans.

So, what was I to do about it? Studying the relevant literature in the field of language assessment and beyond, I quickly learned two lessons: First, rater variability of the kind observed in the context of our new language test, the TestDaF (Test of German as a Foreign Language), is a notorious problem that has always plagued human ratings. Second, at least part of the problem has a solution, and this solution builds on a Rasch measurement approach.

Having been trained in psychometrics and multivariate statistics, I was drawn to the many-facet Rasch measurement (MFRM) model advanced by Linacre (1989). It appeared to me that this model could provide the answer to the question of how to deal appropriately with the error-proneness of human ratings. Yet, it was not until October 2002, when I attended a workshop on many-facet Rasch measurement conducted by Dr. Linacre in Chicago, that I made up my mind to use this model operationally with the TestDaF writing and speaking sections. Back home in Germany, it took a while to convince those in charge of our testing program of the unique advantages offered by MFRM. But in the end I received broad support for implementing this innovative approach. It has been in place now for a number of years, and it has been working just fine.

In a sense, then, this book covers much of what I have learned about MFRM from using it on a routine basis. Hence, the book is written from an applied perspective: It introduces basic concepts, analytical procedures, and statistical methods needed in constructing proficiency measures based on human ratings of examinee performance. Each book chapter thus serves to corroborate the famous dictum that "there is nothing more practical than a good theory" (Lewin, 1951, p. 169). Though the focus of the MFRM applications presented herein is on language assessment, the basic principles readily generalize to any instance of rater-mediated performance assessment typically found in the broader fields of education, employment, the health sciences, and many others.

The present book emerged from an invited chapter included in the *Reference Supplement* to the Manual for *Relating Language Examinations to the Common European Framework of Reference for Languages* (CEFR; Council of Europe, 2009), Section H (Eckes, 2009a). Once more, I would like to thank the members of the Council of Europe's Manual Authoring Group, Brian North, Sauli Takala (editor of the Reference Supplement), and Norman D. Verhelst, for helpful comments and suggestions on earlier drafts of that chapter. In addition, I received valuable feedback on the chapter from Rüdiger Grotjahn, Klaus D. Kubinger, J. Michael Linacre, and Carol M. Myford. When the chapter had evolved into this introduction, I was lucky enough to receive again feedback on the completely revised and expanded text, or parts of it, from Mike Linacre and Carol Myford. I highly appreciate their support and encouragement during my preoccupation with some of the more intricate and challenging issues of the MFRM approach. Of course, any remaining errors and shortcomings are mine.

I would also like to express my gratitude to my colleagues at the TestDaF Institute, Bochum, Germany, for many stimulating discussions concerning the design, analysis, and evaluation of writing and speaking performance assessments. Special thanks go to Achim Althaus, Director of the TestDaF Institute, who greatly supported me in striking a new path for designing a high-quality system of performance ratings. The editors of the series *Language Testing and Evaluation*, Rüdiger Grotjahn and Günther Sigott, warmly welcomed my book proposal. Sarah Kunert and Miriam Matenia, research assistants at the TestDaF Institute, helped with preparing the author and subject indexes.

Last, but not least, I would like to thank those persons close to me. My wife Andrea encouraged me to get the project started and provided the support to keep going. My children Laura and Miriam shared with me their experiences of rater variability at school (though they would not call it that), grumbling about Math teachers being unreasonably severe and others overly lenient, or about English teachers eagerly counting mistakes and others focusing on the skillful use of idiomatic expressions, to mention just a few examples. Looking back at my own schooldays, it is tempting to conclude that rater variability at school is one of the most reliable things in life. At the same time, this recurring variability pushed my motivation for finishing the book project to ever higher levels.

Indeed, my prime goal of writing this book was to introduce those who in some way or another employ, oversee, or evaluate rater-mediated performance assessments to the functionality and practical utility of many-facet Rasch measurement. To the extent that readers feel stimulated to adopt the MFRM approach in their own professional context, this goal has been achieved. So, finally, these are times of hope and confidence.

Thomas Eckes
March, 2011

Preface to the Second Edition

This second edition of my *Introduction to Many-Facet Rasch Measurement* is an extensive revision of the earlier book. I have been motivated by the many positive reactions from readers, and by learning that researchers and practitioners across wide-ranging fields of application are more than ever ready to address the perennial problems inherent in rater-mediated assessments building on a many-facet Rasch measurement approach.

In the present edition, I have revised and updated each chapter, expanded most chapters, and added a completely new chapter. Here I provide a brief outline of the major changes: Chapter 2 ("Rasch Measurement: The Basics") discusses more deeply the fundamental, dichotomous Rasch model, elaborating on key terms such as latent variable, item information, and measurement invariance. Chapter 5 ("A Closer Look at the Rater Facet") has been reorganized, dealing in a separate section with rater severity estimates and their precision; the section on rater fit statistics now includes a detailed discussion of the sample size issue. Further major amendments concern Chapter 6 ("Analyzing the Examinee Facet"), with new sections on examinee measurement results, examinee fit statistics, and criterion-specific score adjustment, and Chapter 7 ("Criteria and Scale Categories"), with new sections on criterion measurement results, manifest and latent rating scale structures, and indicators of rating scale quality. Chapter 8 ("Advanced Many-Facet Rasch Measurement"), probes more deeply into methods of confirmatory interaction analysis, focusing on approaches using dummy facets. The book now closes with Chapter 10 ("Summary and Conclusions"). In this chapter, I recapitulate relevant steps and procedures to consider when conducting a many-facet Rasch analysis, briefly discuss MFRM studies in a number of different fields of application, reconsider the implications of many-facet Rasch measurement for the validity and fairness of inferences drawn from assessment outcomes, and highlight the use of MFRM models within the context of mixed methods approaches to examining raters' cognitive and decision-making processes.

I would like to thank my colleagues at the TestDaF Institute, University of Bochum, Germany, for keeping me attuned to the practical implications of many-facet Rasch measurement within a high-stakes assessment context. I am also grateful to research assistants Anastasia Bobukh-Weiß and Katharina Sokolski who diligently updated the author and subject indexes. My special thanks are due to Carol Myford and Mike Linacre who once more took their time to provide me with valuable feedback on this revised edition. As before, the errors that may remain are entirely my own.

The many-facet extension of the basic, dichotomous Rasch model ensures real progress by enhancing the validity and fairness of rater-mediated assessments across a steadily growing number of disciplines. Hopefully, this book will continue to play its part in further disseminating the rationale and practical utility of many-facet Rasch measurement.

Thomas Eckes
May, 2015

1. Introduction

This chapter introduces the basic idea of many-facet Rasch measurement. Three examples of assessment procedures taken from the field of language testing illustrate the broader context of its application. In the first example, examinees respond to items of a reading comprehension test. The second example refers to a writing performance assessment, where raters evaluate the quality of essays. In the third example, raters evaluate the performance of examinees on a speaking assessment involving live interviewers. Having discussed key concepts such as *facets* and *rater-mediated assessment*, the general steps involved in adopting a many-facet Rasch measurement approach are pointed out. The chapter concludes with an outline of the book's purpose and a brief overview of the chapters to come.

1.1 Facets of measurement

The field of language testing and assessment traditionally draws on a large and diverse set of procedures that aim at measuring a person's language ability or some aspect of that ability (e.g., Alderson & Banerjee, 2001, 2002; Bachman & Palmer, 1996; Spolsky, 1995). For example, in a reading comprehension test examinees may be asked to read a short text and respond to a number of questions or items that relate to the text by selecting the correct answer from several options given. Examinee responses to items may be scored either correct or incorrect according to a well-defined key. Assuming that the test measures what it is intended to measure, that is, when the number-correct score can be interpreted in terms of an examinee's reading ability, the probability of getting a particular item correct will depend on that ability and the difficulty of the item.

In another procedure, examinees are presented with several writing tasks and asked to write short essays summarizing information or discussing issues stated in the tasks. Each essay may be scored by trained raters using a single, holistic rating scale. Here, an examinee's chances of getting a high score on a particular task will depend not only on his or her writing ability and the difficulty of the task, but also on various characteristics of the raters, such as individual raters' tendency to assign overly harsh or lenient ratings, or their general preference for using the middle categories of the rating scale. Moreover, the nature of the rating scale itself is an issue. Thus, the scale categories, or the performance levels they represent, may be defined in a way that makes it hard for an examinee to get a high score.

As a third example, consider a foreign language face-to-face interview where a live interviewer elicits responses from an examinee employing a number of speaking tasks that gradually increase in difficulty level. Each spoken response is recorded on disk and scored by raters according to a set of distinct criteria (e.g., comprehensibility, content, vocabulary, etc.). In this case, the list of variables that may affect the scores finally awarded to examinees is yet longer than in the writing assessment example. Relevant variables include examinee speaking ability, the difficulty of the speaking tasks, the difficulty (or challenge) that the interviewer's style of interaction presents for the examinee, the severity or leniency of the raters, the difficulty of the rating criteria, and the difficulty of the rating scale categories.

The first example, the reading comprehension test, describes a frequently encountered measurement situation involving two components or facets: examinees and test items. Technically speaking, each individual examinee is an element of the *examinee facet*, and each individual test item is an element of the *item facet*. Defined in terms of the measurement variables that are assumed to be relevant in this context, the ability (or proficiency, competence) of an examinee interacts with the difficulty of an item to produce an observed response (the terms *ability*, *proficiency*, or *competence* will be used interchangeably in this book).

The second example, the essay writing, is typical of a situation called *rater-mediated assessment* (Engelhard, 2002; McNamara, 2000), also known as a *performance test* (McNamara, 1996; Wigglesworth, 2008) or *performance assessment* (Johnson, Penny, & Gordon, 2009; Lane & Stone, 2006). In rater-mediated assessment, one more facet is added to the set of facets that may have an impact on examinee scores (besides the examinee and task facets)—the *rater facet*. As discussed in detail later, the rater facet is unduly influential in many circumstances. Specifically, raters (also called graders, markers, scorers, readers, or judges) often constitute an important source of variation in observed (or raw) scores that is unwanted because it threatens the validity of the inferences drawn from assessment outcomes.

The last example, the face-to-face interview, is similarly an instance of rater-mediated assessment, but represents a situation of significantly heightened complexity. At least five facets, and possibly various interactions among them, can be assumed to have an impact on the measurement results. These facets, in particular examinees, tasks, interviewers, scoring criteria, and raters, in some way or other codetermine the scores finally awarded to examinees' spoken performance.

As the examples demonstrate, assessment situations are characterized by distinct sets of factors directly or indirectly involved in bringing about measurement outcomes. More generally speaking, a *facet* can be defined as any factor, variable, or component of the measurement situation that is assumed to affect test or assessment scores in a systematic way (Bachman, 2004; Linacre, 2002a; Wolfe & Dobria, 2008). This definition includes facets that are of substantive interest (e.g., examinees), as well as facets that are assumed to contribute systematic measurement error (e.g., raters, tasks, criteria, interviewers, time of testing). Moreover, facets can interact with each other in various ways. For instance, elements of one facet (e.g., individual raters) may differentially influence scores when paired with subsets of elements of another facet (e.g., female or male examinees). Besides two-way interactions, higher-order interactions among particular elements, or subsets of elements, of three or more facets may also come into play and affect scores in subtle, yet systematic ways.

The error-prone nature of most measurement facets, in particular the fallibility of human raters, raises serious concerns regarding the psychometric quality of the scores awarded to examinees. These concerns need to be addressed carefully, particularly in high-stakes assessments, the results of which heavily influence examinees' career or study plans. As discussed throughout this book, many facets other than those associated with the construct being measured can have a non-negligible impact on the outcomes of assessment procedures. Therefore, the construction of reliable, valid, and fair measures of examinee ability depends crucially on the implementation of well-designed methods to deal with multiple sources of variability that characterize many-facet assessment situations.

Viewed from a measurement perspective, an adequate approach to the analysis of many-facet data would involve three general steps as shown in Figure 1.1. These steps form the methodological basis of a measurement approach to the analysis and evaluation of performance assessments, in particular rater-mediated assessments.

Fig. 1.1: Basic three-step measurement approach to the analysis and evaluation of performance assessments.

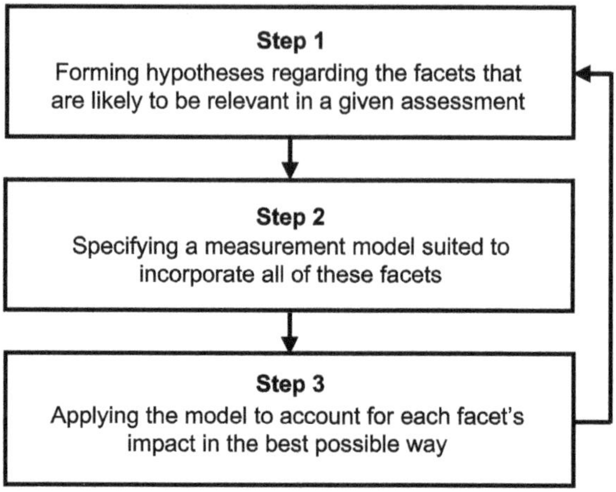

Step 1 starts with a careful inspection of the overall design and the development of the assessment procedure. Issues to be considered at this stage include defining the group of examinees at which the assessment is targeted, selecting the raters, and determining the scoring approach (number and kind of scoring criteria, number of performance tasks, scale categories, etc.). This step is completed when the facets have been identified that can be assumed to have an impact on the assessment. Usually there is a small set of key facets that are considered on a routine basis (e.g., examinees, raters, criteria, tasks). Yet, as explained later, this set of facets may not be exhaustive in the sense that other, less obvious facets could have an additional effect.

Steps 2 and 3, respectively, address the choice and implementation of a reasonable psychometric model. Specifying such a model will give an operational answer to the question of what facets are likely to come into play in the assessment process; applying the model will provide insight into the adequacy of the overall measurement approach, the accuracy of the measures constructed, and the validity of the inferences made from those measures. As indicated by the arrow leading back from Step 3 to Step 1, the measurement outcomes may also serve to modify the hypotheses on which the model specified in Step 2 was based or to form new hypotheses that better represent the set of facets having an impact on the assessment. This book deals mainly with Steps 2 and 3.

1.2 Purpose and plan of the book

In this book, I present an approach to the measurement of examinee proficiency that is particularly well-suited to dealing with many-facet data typically generated in rater-mediated assessments. In particular, I give an introductory overview of a general psychometric modeling approach called *many-facet Rasch measurement* (MFRM). This term goes back to Linacre (1989). Other commonly used terms are, for example, *multi-facet(ed)* or *many-faceted Rasch measurement* (Engelhard, 1992, 1994; McNamara, 1996), *many-faceted conjoint measurement* (Linacre, Engelhard, Tatum, & Myford, 1994), or *multifacet Rasch modeling* (Lunz & Linacre, 1998).

My focus in the book is on the rater facet and its various ramifications. Raters are almost indispensable in assessing performance on tasks that require examinees to create a response. Such tasks range from limited production tasks like short-answer questions to extended production tasks that prompt examinees to write an essay, deliver a speech, or provide work samples (Carr, 2011; Johnson et al., 2009). The generic term for these kinds of tasks is *constructed-response tasks*, as opposed to *selected-response tasks*, where examinees are to choose the correct answer from a number of alternatives given. Typical selected-response task formats include multiple-choice or true–false items.

This book heavily draws on a field of application where raters have always figured prominently: the assessment of language performance, particularly with respect to the productive skills of writing and speaking. Since the "communicative turn" in language testing, starting around the late 1970s (e.g., Bachman, 2000; McNamara, 1996, 2014; Morrow, 1979), raters have played an increasingly important role. Yet, from the very beginning, rating quality studies have pointed to a wide range of rater errors and biases (e.g., Guilford, 1936; Hoyt, 2000; Kingsbury, 1922; Saal, Downey, & Lahey, 1980; Wind & Engelhard, 2013). For example, it may be known that some raters tend to assign lower ratings than others to the very same performance; when these raters are to evaluate examinee performance in an operational setting, luck of the draw can unfairly affect assessment outcomes. As will be shown, MFRM provides a rich set of highly efficient tools to account, and compensate, for rater-dependent measurement error.

The book is organized as follows. In the next chapter, Chapter 2, I briefly describe the principles of Rasch measurement and discuss implications of choosing a Rasch modeling approach to the analysis of many-facet data. Chapter 3 deals with the challenge that rater-mediated assessment poses to assuring high-quality ratings. In particular, I probe into the issue of rater error. The traditional or standard approach to dealing with rater error is to train raters, to compute an index of interrater reliability, and to show that the agreement among raters is sufficiently high. However, in many instances this approach is strongly limited. In order to discuss some of the possible shortcomings and pitfalls, I draw on a sample data set taken from a live assessment of foreign-language writing performance. For the purposes of widening the perspective, I go on describing a conceptual–psychometric framework incorporating multiple kinds of facets that potentially have an impact on the process of rating examinee performance on writing tasks.

In keeping with Step 1 outlined above (Figure 1.1), the potentially relevant facets need to be identified first. Incorporating these facets into a many-facet Rasch measurement (MFRM) model will allow the researcher to closely examine each of the facets and their interrelationships (Step 2). To illustrate the application of such a model (Step 3), I draw again on the writing data and show how that model can be used to gain insight into the many-facet nature of the data (Chapter 4). In Chapters 5 and 6, I pay particular attention to the rater and examinee facets, respectively. In Chapter 7, the discussion focuses on the way raters use the scoring criteria and the different categories of the rating scale.

Chapter 8 illustrates the versatility of the MFRM approach by presenting a number of more advanced models that can be used for analyzing multiple kinds of data and for studying various interactions between facets. The chapter closes with a summary presentation of commonly used models suitable for evaluating the psychometric quality of many-facet data.

Chapter 9 addresses special issues of some practical concern, such as choosing an appropriate rating design, providing informative feedback to raters, and using many-facet Rasch measurement for standard-setting purposes. On a more theoretical note, I deal with differences between MFRM modeling and generalizability theory (G-theory), a psychometric approach rooted in classical test theory that takes different sources of measurement error into account. Finally, I briefly discuss computer programs currently available for conducting a many-facet Rasch analysis, including some extensions of the MFRM approach.

The last chapter, Chapter 10, first provides a summary of major steps and procedures of a standard many-facet Rasch analysis and then presents illustrative MFRM studies drawn from wide-ranging fields of application. After discussing the relationship between measurement and issues of validating performance assessments more generally, the focus shifts toward the potential contribution of MFRM to investigations of rater cognition issues building on mixed methods research designs.

2. Rasch Measurement: The Basics

Many-facet Rasch measurement models belong to a whole family of models that have their roots in the dichotomous Rasch model (Rasch, 1960/1980). Rasch models share assumptions that set them apart from other psychometric approaches often used for the analysis and evaluation of tests and assessments. To better understand what the distinctive properties of Rasch models are and how many-facet Rasch measurement models differ from the standard, dichotomous Rasch model, the dichotomous model is presented first. Then, two extensions of the model are briefly discussed that are suited for the analysis of rating data. The final section introduces the sample data that will be considered throughout the book to illustrate the rationale and practical use of many-facet Rasch measurement.

2.1 Elements of Rasch measurement

2.1.1 The dichotomous Rasch model

Consider again the first introductory example of language assessment procedures. This example referred to a reading comprehension test that employed a multiple-choice format; that is, the examinees were asked to respond to reading items by selecting the correct option from a number of alternatives given. Responses to each item were scored either correct or incorrect. In such a case, each item has exactly two possible, mutually exclusive score categories. Items exhibiting this kind of two-category or binary format are called *dichotomous* items. Usually, an examinee's score on such a test is the number-correct score, computed as the number of items that the examinee answered correctly.

Rasch (1960/1980)[1] developed a measurement model for responses to dichotomous items. This model has been variously referred to as the *Rasch model* (e.g., Wright & Stone, 1979), the *basic* or *dichotomous Rasch model* (e.g., Wright &

1 Georg Rasch (1901–1980) was a Danish mathematician and statistician. For a detailed account of Rasch's life and work, see Andersen and Olsen (2001; see also Andersen, 1982; Andrich, 2005a). Insightful views of early personal encounters with Rasch and his revolutionary ideas have been provided by two scholars who themselves greatly contributed to disseminating around the world Rasch's approach to measurement, Gerhard H. Fischer (University of Vienna, Austria; Fischer, 2010) and Benjamin D. Wright (University of Chicago, IL; Wright & Andrich, 1987).

Masters, 1982), the *simple logistic model* (e.g., Andrich, 1988), or the *one-parameter logistic (1PL) model* (e.g., Yen & Fitzpatrick, 2006). The literature dealing with the model and its extensions has been growing rapidly over the years. Hence, this section focuses on key concepts and principles needed for a basic understanding of Rasch measurement. For more detailed discussions, the reader is referred to textbooks on Rasch models and related psychometric approaches (e.g., Bond & Fox, 2015; Boone, Staver, & Yale, 2014; de Ayala, 2009; DeMars, 2010; Embretson & Reise, 2000; Engelhard, 2013; Wilson, 2005).

The following equation defines the dichotomous Rasch model:

$$p(x_{ni} = 1) = \frac{\exp(\theta_n - \beta_i)}{1 + \exp(\theta_n - \beta_i)}, \tag{2.1}$$

where x_{ni} is the score of examinee n for item i, with $x_{ni} = 1$ for a correct response and $x_{ni} = 0$ for an incorrect response; θ_n is the ability of examinee n; β_i is the difficulty of item i.

Equation 2.1 presents the dichotomous Rasch model in its exponential form. As usual, $\exp(\theta_n - \beta_i)$ denotes e, the base of the natural logarithm (e is approximately equal to 2.7183), raised to the power $(\theta_n - \beta_i)$.

According to this model, the probability that examinee n answers item i correctly, that is, $p(x_{ni} = 1)$, depends on the difference between the ability of the examinee (θ_n) and the difficulty of the item (β_i). Thus, if an examinee's ability equals an item's difficulty, that is, if $\theta_n - \beta_i = 0$, with $\exp(0) = 1$, the examinee has a .50 chance of getting the item correct.

In measurement contexts, the term *ability* is typically used in a broad, generic sense, referring to a *latent variable* that represents the construct of interest. The variable is called "latent" because it is not directly observable but manifests itself in observable responses. These responses may be answers of examinees to items or scores that raters award to an examinee's performance on a task. In terms of a spatial metaphor, the latent variable is also called a *latent dimension* or *latent continuum*.

Fig. 2.1: Item characteristic curves for three items under the dichotomous Rasch model.

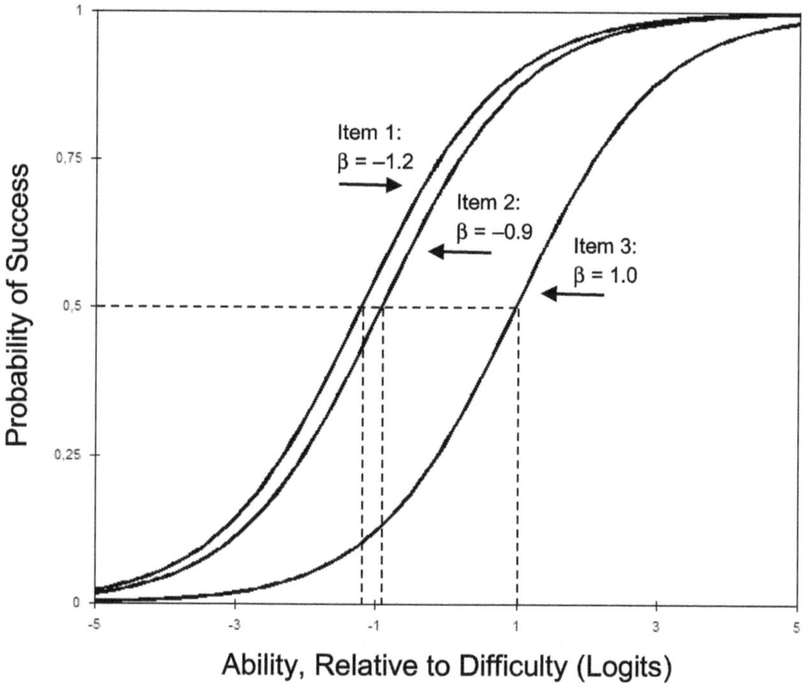

The mathematical function shown in Equation 2.1 is an example of a *logistic function*: For any given item *i*, the probability of a correct response (success of examinee *n* on item *i*) increases strictly monotonically with increasing levels of ability. This functional relationship can be described by an S-shaped curve, a *logistic ogive*, also known as an *item characteristic curve* (ICC) or *item response function* (IRF). Figure 2.1 displays the ICCs for three items according to the dichotomous Rasch model. Each curve (solid line) represents one item.

The probability of success on an item is shown along the vertical axis, ranging from 0 to 1; the ability levels (θ values) are shown along the horizontal axis. More specifically, the horizontal axis represents the latent dimension; that is, it represents examinee ability relative to item difficulty ($\theta_n - \beta_i$). As explained in more detail later, the measurement units of this dimension are shown in logits, ranging from minus infinity (−∞) to plus infinity (+∞). For ease of presentation, θ values are displayed within a bounded range of −5.0 to 5.0 logits. Figure 2.1 shows that the probability of success on an item approaches 0 for very low ability levels and approaches 1 for very high ability levels.

The difficulty of an item is commonly defined as the level of examinee ability at which the probability of a correct response is .50 (the horizontal dashed line in Figure 2.1 is drawn at this probability value). As indicated by the vertical dashed lines, Item 1 is slightly easier than Item 2, which in turn is much easier than Item 3. Put differently, Item 1 requires the least amount of ability to be answered correctly; Item 3 requires the highest amount of ability: Only examinees with ability greater than 1 logit have a probability of getting Item 3 correct greater than .50.

The slope of each ICC is highest when the ability level equals an item's difficulty. It is exactly at this location on the latent dimension that the *uncertainty* about an examinee's response is highest: there is a 50% chance that the examinee will succeed on the item and a 50% chance that the examinee will fail on the item. For an examinee with ability 2.2 logits higher than an item's difficulty, the degree of uncertainty is greatly reduced: the probability of success is 90%. In other words, the item is much too easy for the examinee; it provides only little information about the examinee's relative standing on the latent dimension. Specifically, if $\theta_n - \beta_i = 2.2$, the *item information* is $p(x_{ni} = 1)p(x_{ni} = 0) = .90(.10) = .09$. The item information reaches its maximum value, if $\theta_n = \beta_i$, which is $.50(.50) = .25$.

Examinee ability and item difficulty (Equation 2.1) are model parameters. These have to be estimated from empirical observations, for example, from responses of examinees to items. There are a number of different estimation algorithms available, a discussion of which is beyond the scope of the present introduction (e.g., Baker & Kim, 2004; Wright & Masters, 1982; Yen & Fitzpatrick, 2006; for a brief outline, see Section 9.5 on MFRM software). Estimation of parameters is sometimes called *calibration*.

The basic Rasch model specifies a single item parameter, that is, item difficulty; hence the occasionally found designation as "1PL model". Most importantly, Rasch models share the assumption that all items have identical discrimination (fixed at 1.0); that is, for all items the ICCs are assumed to be *parallel*, non-intersecting curves, differing only in their location on the latent dimension. As a result, the ordering of items by difficulty is the same for all ability levels. It also follows that the ordering of examinees by ability is the same for all difficulty levels; that is, regardless of which item is encountered, an examinee who is more able has a higher chance of success than an examinee who is less able. This assumption establishes the fundamental Rasch model property of *measurement invariance* or *specific objectivity* (Bond & Fox, 2015; DeMars, 2010; Engelhard, 2013; Iramaneerat, Smith, & Smith, 2008). Note that measurement invariance is a property of models belonging to the family of Rasch models; it is only a property of data, if the data fit a given Rasch model.

An alternative expression of the dichotomous Rasch model is in terms of *log odds*. Odds are defined as a ratio of the number of successes to the number of failures. Thus, if the odds that an examinee answers an item correctly are 4/1, then out of five attempts, four successes (i.e., correct answers) and one failure (i.e., incorrect answer) are expected. Put differently, odds are the probability of success divided by the probability of failure. In the example, the probability of success is .80 and the probability of failure is .20; that is, the odds are .80/.20.

To derive the log odds form of the Rasch model, the probability that examinee n answers item i correctly, $p(x_{ni} = 1)$, is divided by the probability that examinee n answers item i incorrectly, $p(x_{ni} = 0)$:

$$\frac{p(x_{ni}=1)}{p(x_{ni}=0)} = \exp(\theta_n - \beta_i). \tag{2.2}$$

Taking the natural logarithm of the odds ratio yields the log odds form of the dichotomous Rasch model:

$$\ln\left[\frac{p(x_{ni}=1)}{p(x_{ni}=0)}\right] = \theta_n - \beta_i. \tag{2.3}$$

The natural logarithm of the odds ratio is called *logit*, which is short for "log odds unit". Under this model, the logit is a simple linear function of the ability parameter θ_n and the difficulty parameter β_i. Clearly, when the examinee ability equals the item difficulty, the log odds of success are zero.

The measurement scale that defines the horizontal (latent) dimension in Figure 2.1 is the *logit scale*. Both examinee ability and item difficulty are expressed on this scale. Generally, the logit is the *measurement unit* of the scale for any parameter specified in a Rasch model. Considering the model shown in Equation 2.3, one logit is the distance along the measurement scale that increases the odds of success by a factor of approximately 2.7183, the value of *e* (see Linacre & Wright, 1989; Ludlow & Haley, 1995).

When the data fit the Rasch model, the logit measures are on an interval scale. Therefore, Rasch models are suited to constructing linear measures from counts of qualitatively ordered observations (e.g., number-correct scores, performance ratings).

Besides the construction of interval measures, Rasch models have distinct advantages over related psychometric approaches that have been proposed in an item response theory (IRT) framework (for an overview of IRT models, see, e.g., de Ayala, 2009; DeMars, 2010; Yen & Fitzpatrick, 2006). The most important advantage has already been mentioned: measurement invariance. Thus, when a given set of observations fits the Rasch model, examinee measures are invariant across different sets of items (i.e., examinee measures are "item-free" or "test-free") and item measures are invariant across different groups of examinees (i.e., item measures are "examinee-free" or "sample-free"; Wright, 1967, 1999).

The log odds form of the Rasch model (Equation 2.3) can be used to demonstrate the invariance property. Consider two examinees with abilities θ_1 and θ_2 responding to an item with difficulty β_i. The log odds for these two examinees are as follows:

$$\ln\left[\frac{p(x_{1i}=1)}{p(x_{1i}=0)}\right]=\theta_1-\beta_i \tag{2.4}$$

and

$$\ln\left[\frac{p(x_{2i}=1)}{p(x_{2i}=0)}\right]=\theta_2-\beta_i. \tag{2.5}$$

The difference between the log odds is given by

$$\ln\left[\frac{p(x_{1i}=1)}{p(x_{1i}=0)}\right]-\ln\left[\frac{p(x_{2i}=1)}{p(x_{2i}=0)}\right]=\theta_1-\beta_i-(\theta_2-\beta_i)=\theta_1-\theta_2. \tag{2.6}$$

Equation 2.6 shows that the difference between the log odds for two examinees depends only on the examinees' ability parameters and not on the item parameter. That is, irrespective of which items are used to compare the examinees, the difference between the log odds for the examinees is the same. Likewise, it can be demonstrated that the comparison between two items is "examinee-free". That is, the difference between the log odds for two items is the same regardless of which examinee answered the two items (see also Schmidt & Embretson, 2003; Woods & Baker, 1985).

Measurement invariance has an important implication: Test scores are *sufficient statistics* for the estimation of examinee ability; that is, the number-correct score contains all the information required for the estimation of an examinee's measure from a given set of observations. In other words, it does not matter *which* items an examinee answered correctly; all that counts is *how many* items the examinee answered correctly. The same holds true for the estimation of item difficulty: Only relevant for the estimation of an item's measure is how many examinees answered that item correctly. By contrast, IRT models like the *two-parameter logistic* (2PL) model (incorporating item difficulty and item discrimination parameters) or the *three-parameter logistic* (3PL) model (incorporating a guessing parameter in addition to item difficulty and discrimination parameters) lack the property of measurement invariance; parameter estimation, therefore, does not rest on sufficient statistics (Andrich, 2004; Kubinger, 2005; Wright, 1999). These models are not considered further in this book.

Two properties that Rasch models share with many IRT models commonly in use are *unidimensional* measurement and *local (conditional) independence*. Items that conform to Rasch model assumptions measure one latent variable; that is, no other variables or dimensions are involved (Engelhard, 2013; Fischer, 1995a; Henning, 1992). Local independence implies that an examinee's response to an item does not affect the probability of the examinee's response to another item: The joint probability of two item responses is equal to the product of the individual probabilities of the two item responses, conditional on the latent variable being measured (Fischer, 1995a; Henning, 1989; Yen & Fitzpatrick, 2006).

2.1.2 Polytomous Rasch models

In the following, I briefly discuss two widely used extensions of the dichotomous Rasch model that are of particular importance to a many-facet Rasch measurement approach. Both extensions are designed for modeling *polytomous items*; that is, items with more than two (inherently ordered) response categories. Typically, ordered polytomous data result from the use of rating scales. For example, when measuring social attitudes four-category Likert-type scales are commonly used, with categories such as *strongly disagree*, *disagree*, *agree*, and *strongly agree*. Polytomous Rasch models add parameters to the basic Rasch model that describe the functioning of the rating scale (e.g., Andrich, 2005b; Embretson & Reise, 2000; Ostini & Nering, 2006; Penfield, 2014).

The first polytomous Rasch model considered here is the *rating scale model* (RSM; Andrich, 1978; see also Andersen, 2005). The RSM adds a threshold parameter to represent the relative difficulty of a transition from one category of the rating scale to the next.

Specifically, the *threshold parameter*, or *category coefficient*, τ_k, is the location on the latent dimension where the adjacent categories, k and $k - 1$, are equally probable to be observed. In other words, τ_k represents the transition point at which the probability is 50% of an examinee responding in one of two adjacent categories, given that the examinee is in one of those two categories. These transition points are called *Rasch-Andrich thresholds* (Bond & Fox, 2015; Linacre, 2006a, 2010b; see also Andrich, 1998, 2005b).

The log odds form of the RSM is given by

$$\ln\left[\frac{p_{nik}}{p_{nik-1}}\right] = \theta_n - \beta_i - \tau_k, \tag{2.7}$$

where p_{nik} is the probability that an examinee n responds with category k to item i; p_{nik-1} is the probability that an examinee n responds with category $k - 1$ to item i; k is a response category of a rating scale that has $m + 1$ categories (i.e., $k = 0, \ldots, m$); τ_k is the difficulty of responding with category k (relative to $k - 1$). The difficulty of a polytomous item i, β_i, is defined as the location on the latent dimension where the lowest and highest categories are equally probable.

The RSM assumes the same set of threshold parameters across all items (or rating scales) on the test. Therefore, the model should only be used when the items have a common rating scale structure; that is, when the items have the same number of response categories, and the relative difficulty between categories is constant across the items.

When the items have different numbers of response categories or when the relative difficulty between categories is expected to vary from item to item, the *partial credit model* (PCM; Masters, 1982, 2010) is a suitable alternative. The PCM estimates threshold parameters for each item separately, allowing each item to have a unique rating scale structure. The log odds form of the PCM is given by

$$\ln\left[\frac{p_{nik}}{p_{nik-1}}\right] = \theta_n - \beta_i - \tau_{ik}, \tag{2.8}$$

where p_{nik} is the probability that an examinee n responds with category k to item i; p_{nik-1} is the probability that an examinee n responds with category $k - 1$ to item i; k is a response category of a rating scale that has $m_i + 1$ categories (i.e., $k = 0, \ldots, m_i$); τ_{ik} is the difficulty of responding with category k to item i (relative to $k - 1$).

2.2 Rasch modeling of many-facet data

Many-facet Rasch measurement refers to a class of measurement models suitable for a simultaneous analysis of multiple variables potentially having an impact on assessment outcomes. MFRM models, also known as *facets models*, incorporate more variables, or facets, than the two that are included in a classical testing situation. As the introductory examples have shown, performance assessments typically include not only examinee and item (or task) facets, but also other facets such as raters, scoring criteria, interviewers and possibly many more.

Facets models belong to the family of Rasch models, including the RSM and the PCM discussed above, the linear logistic test model (LLTM; Fischer, 1973, 1995b, 2005; Kubinger, 2009), the mixed Rasch model (Rost, 1990, 2004), and others (for a detailed discussion, see Fischer, 2007; see also Rost, 2001; Wright & Mok, 2004). Early proposals to extend the basic Rasch model by simultaneously taking into account three or more facets ("experimental factors") were made by Micko (1969, 1970) and Kempf (1972). Note also that Linacre's (1989) MFRM modeling approach can be considered a special case of Fischer's (1973) LLTM (e.g., Kline, Schmidt, Bowles, 2006; Linacre, 2002a; Rost & Langeheine, 1997).

Since its first comprehensive theoretical statement (Linacre, 1989), many-facet Rasch measurement has been used in a rapidly increasing number of substantive applications in the fields of language testing, educational and psychological measurement, the health sciences, and many others (e.g., Barkaoui, 2014; Bond & Fox, 2015; Engelhard, 2002, 2013). Section 10.2 covers a broad range of illustrative MFRM studies, highlighting its practical utility in different applied settings.

As a prominent example from the field of applied linguistics, MFRM has been decisive for the development of the descriptor scales advanced by the Common European Framework of Reference for Languages (CEFR; Council of Europe, 2001; see also North, 2000, 2008; North & Jones, 2009; North & Schneider, 1998). In addition, the MFRM approach has provided the methodological basis for preparing illustrative CEFR samples of spoken production for English, French, German, and Italian (Breton, Lepage, & North, 2008). Thus, as North (2000, p. 349) put it, many-facet Rasch measurement has been "uniquely relevant to the development of a common framework". More generally, pointing to the close interrelations between applied linguistics and measurement, McNamara (2011, pp. 436–437) noted that MFRM has become "a standard part of the training of language testers, and is routinely used in research on performance assessment" (see also McNamara & Knoch, 2012).

In what follows, I first pick up again on the second and third introductory examples of language assessment procedures. Then, I introduce the sample data that will be used for the purposes of illustration throughout the book.

2.2.1 Putting the facets together

In an assessment situation involving raters using a single rating scale (e.g., a four-category scale) to evaluate globally the quality of examinee performance there are at least two facets to be distinguished, raters and examinees. If examinees respond to each of a number of tasks, and raters provide ratings of examinee performance on each task separately, then the task facet also needs to be considered. That is, examinees, tasks, and raters define a three-facet situation of the kind already referred to in the second introductory example of language assessment procedures.

Presupposing that the relevant facets have been identified (i.e., examinees, tasks, and raters), a suitable many-facet Rasch measurement model may be formally expressed like this:

$$\ln\left[\frac{p_{nljk}}{p_{nljk-1}}\right] = \theta_n - \delta_l - \alpha_j - \tau_k, \qquad (2.9)$$

where

p_{nijk} = probability of examinee *n* receiving a rating of *k* from rater *j* on task *l*,
p_{nijk-1} = probability of examinee *n* receiving a rating of *k* – 1 from rater *j* on task *l*,
θ_n = ability of examinee *n*,
δ_l = difficulty of task *l*,
α_j = severity of rater *j*,
τ_k = difficulty of receiving a rating of *k* relative to *k* – 1.

As shown in Equation 2.9, a MFRM model is essentially an additive-linear model that is based on a logistic transformation of observed ratings to a logit scale ("additive" here means "combined by the rules of addition and subtraction"). Using standard statistical terminology (e.g., Hays, 1994; Myers, Well, & Lorch, 2010), the logistic transformation of ratios of successive category probabilities (i.e., log odds) can be viewed as the *dependent variable* with various facets, such as examinees, tasks, and raters, conceptualized as *independent variables* that influence these log odds.

The threshold parameter, τ_k, indicates how the rating data are to be handled. In Equation 2.9, the parameter specifies that a RSM should be used across all elements of each facet. For example, in the analysis, the four-category scale is treated as if all raters understood and used each rating scale category in a highly similar manner. Regarding the task facet this means that a particular rating, such as "2" on Task 1, is assumed to be equivalent to a rating of "2" on Task 2 and on all the other tasks included in the assessment. More specifically, the threshold parameters are calibrated jointly across raters (and across tasks and examinees); that is, the set of threshold parameters, which defines the *structure* of the rating scale, is the same for all raters (and for all tasks and examinees). Hence, Equation 2.9 is an expression for a *three-facet rating scale model* (Linacre & Wright, 2002). Alternatively, the threshold parameter could be specified in such a way as to allow for variable rating scale structures across elements of a particular facet, implying the use of a *three-facet partial credit model* (Linacre & Wright, 2002; see Section 8.3).

Note the change in meaning of terms used in the three-facet RSM, as compared to the terms used in the original RSM (Equation 2.5). The three-facet RSM does not model an examinee responding with a particular category of the rating scale; rather, this RSM models a rater responding with a particular category of the rating scale based on what he or she believes to characterize the performance of the examinee. Put differently, in Equation 2.9, the threshold parameter, τ_k, does *not* refer to the difficulty of a response in category k (relative to $k - 1$) of the rating scale, but to the difficulty of *receiving* a response in category k (relative to $k - 1$). Thus, it is important to distinguish between the difficulty of showing a response in a particular category and the difficulty of being observed in that category.

More generally, when the data to be modeled refer to ratings, specifying a many-facet RSM (or a many-facet PCM) implies an assumption about how raters make use of the different categories of the rating scale. The key issue can be phrased as follows: Is it reasonable to assume that all raters use the scale in the same way, agreeing upon the performance differences implied by adjacent categories, or is it more likely that some raters follow their own, more or less idiosyncratic style of assigning meaning to the categories?

With increasing professional experience each rater usually comes to adopt a particular approach to the rating task, an approach that may have evolved to work well in the rater's daily work, but that may differ largely from other raters' approaches. Familiarizing raters with the scale to be used surely helps to increase rater agreement in scale usage, but how much can be achieved in any given instance actually remains an open question. Viewed from a measurement perspective, a principled approach to answering this question would involve running a many-facet PCM analysis and comparing the resulting category calibrations across raters.

As shown in Equation 2.9, rater severity is explicitly modeled. Thus, an analysis based on the model provides an estimate of each rater's severity. Generally, *rater severity* is present when raters provide ratings that are consistently too harsh, compared to other raters or to established benchmark ratings (i.e., consensus ratings provided by a group of expert raters for specified levels of examinee ability). Specifically, in Equation 2.9, as in other such model equations discussed later, the parameter α_j models the severity of rater j; that is, the greater the value of this parameter, the lower the rating is predicted to be. Put differently, the model implies that severe or harsh raters tend to award lower scores to examinees, indicating lower examinee ability. Conversely, lenient raters tend to award higher scores. Hence, if one were interested in modeling *rater leniency*, parameter α_j should be added in the model equation (instead of being subtracted).

For cost or efficiency reasons, particularly in the context of large-scale assessments, it is common that not all raters rate the performances of all examinees. Frequently, the assessment design is limited to a double-rating procedure; that is, only two raters out of a larger group of similarly competent raters independently rate the same set of examinee performances. In situations like this, the data matrix containing all the scores awarded to examinees is incomplete; that is, there will be lots of missing data. Provided that the rating design contains sufficient links between the elements of the facets involved, examinee ability, rater severity, and task difficulty parameters, or whatever parameters have been specified in a given model, can still be estimated in a common frame of reference. In other words, Rasch models are robust against missing data since they are only evaluated for observed data points. There is no requirement to impute, or adjust for, unobserved data. In a later chapter (see Section 9.1), various rating designs yielding sparse data matrices that are suited for a many-facet Rasch analysis are discussed more deeply.

Devising an appropriate rating design can become quite a challenging task when more than three facets have been identified. Consider the third introductory example, the live interview. Here, the list of relevant facets includes examinees, tasks, interviewers, scoring criteria, and raters. This translates into the following five-facet rating scale model:

$$\ln\left[\frac{p_{nilvjk}}{p_{nilvjk-1}}\right] = \theta_n - \beta_i - \delta_l - \eta_v - \alpha_j - \tau_k, \tag{2.10}$$

where

p_{nilvjk}	=	probability of examinee n receiving a rating of k from rater j on criterion i for task l presented by interviewer v,
$p_{nilvjk-1}$	=	probability of examinee n receiving a rating of $k - 1$ from rater j on criterion i for task l presented by interviewer v,
θ_n	=	ability of examinee n,
β_i	=	difficulty of criterion i,
δ_l	=	difficulty of task l,
η_v	=	difficulty of interviewer v,
α_j	=	severity of rater j,
τ_k	=	difficulty of receiving a rating of k relative to $k - 1$.

The five-facet RSM (Equation 2.10) concludes this first introductory presentation of MFRM models. Before proceeding to a description of the sample data and the particular MFRM model used to examine these data, the following quotation from the preface of Linacre's (1989) book may serve to highlight the driving forces behind the very development of the MFRM approach to the analysis and evaluation of rater-mediated assessments:

> A conscientious test director realized that the conventional method of basing decisions for rated performances directly on raw scores is unfair to examinees who encounter severe raters. It is also potentially life-threatening when incompetent examinees in some crucial discipline are certified merely because they encounter lenient raters. This realization motivated the question: 'How can fair and meaningful measures be constructed from inevitably dubious ordinal ratings?' MFRM provides the answer. (p. iii)

2.2.2 The sample data: Essay ratings

The data considered throughout this book comprised ratings of examinee performance on the writing section of the Test of German as a Foreign Language (*Test Deutsch als Fremdsprache*, TestDaF). The TestDaF is a standardized test designed for foreign learners of German who plan to study in Germany or who require recognized certification of their language ability. This test was administered worldwide for the first time in April 2001. The live examination considered here took place in October 2001 (for more detail on the TestDaF methodology, see Eckes, 2005b, 2008a, 2010b; see also http://www.testdaf.de).

The writing section assessed an examinee's ability to produce a coherent and well-structured text on a topic taken from the academic context. Examinees were presented with a single complex writing task consisting of two parts. In the first part, charts, tables, or diagrams were provided along with a short introductory text, and the examinee was to describe the relevant information. Specific points to be dealt with were stated in the prompt (the "description part"). In the second part, the examinee had to consider different positions on an aspect of the topic and write a structured argument. The input consisted of short statements, questions, or quotes. As before, aspects to be dealt with were stated in the prompt (the "argumentation part"). Examinees were given 60 minutes to write the essay.

A total of 307 examinees completed the writing task. The essays were evaluated by a total of 18 raters. All raters were specialists in the field of German as a foreign language; raters had been trained and monitored as to compliance with TestDaF scoring guidelines. The number of essays rated by each rater ranged from 19 to 68 ($M = 36.0$, $SD = 13.16$).

Each essay was rated independently by two raters. In addition, one rater provided ratings of two essays that were randomly selected from each of the other 17 raters' workload; that is, there were 34 third ratings. These third ratings served to satisfy the basic requirement of a *connected* data set, where all elements are directly or indirectly linked to each other. Due to this network of links all 18 raters could be directly compared along a single dimension of severity. The connectedness issue is taken up again in Section 9.1 on rating designs.

Ratings were provided on a four-category rating scale printed on a scoring form, with categories labeled by TDN levels (*TestDaF-Niveaustufen*, TDNs). The four scale categories were as follows: *below TDN 3*, *TDN 3*, *TDN 4*, and *TDN 5*. TDN levels 3 to 5 covered the Council of Europe's (2001) Lower Vantage Level (B2.1) to Higher Effective Operational Proficiency (C1.2); that is, the TestDaF measured German language ability at an intermediate to high level (for a detailed study on the ability level implied by each TDN, see Kecker & Eckes, 2010).

Table 2.1: Excerpt from the Essay Rating Sample Data.

		Criterion		
Examinee	**Rater**	**GI**	**TF**	**LR**
001	01	5	5	4
001	14	3	3	3
002	07	4	5	3
002	10	4	4	4
...		.	.	.
...	.	.	.	.
091	08	5	5	5
091	14	4	4	3
092	02	5	4	4
092	04	4	4	4
...	.	.	.	.
...	.	.	.	.
130	07	4	4	3
130	10	4	3	4
131	05	4	2	4
131	06	3	3	3
131	07	4	3	4
...	.	.	.	.
...	.	.	.	.
221	05	3	3	2
221	18	4	3	4
222	03	5	5	5
222	13	5	4	4
...	.	.	.	.
...	.	.	.	.
306	05	3	2	2
306	07	4	3	4
307	11	5	4	5
307	17	5	4	4

Note. GI = global impression. TF = task fulfillment. LR = linguistic realization. Ratings on the TDN scale range from 2 (*below TDN* 3, lowest proficiency level) to 5 (*TDN* 5, highest proficiency level).

Raters evaluated each essay drawing on sets of ordered performance descriptors representing three different criteria. The first criterion referred to *global impression* (a kind of holistic criterion, based on a first reading), encompassing aspects such as fluency, train of thought, and structure; the other two criteria were more of an analytic kind, referring to distinct aspects of *task fulfillment* (i.e., completeness, description, argumentation) and *linguistic realization* (i.e., breadth of syntactic elements, vocabulary, correctness), respectively.

For example, the descriptors for global impression aspect *fluency* were as follows: "The text reads fluently throughout" (*TDN 5*), "Readability is slightly impaired in places" (*TDN 4*), "Repeated reading of parts of the text is necessary" (*TDN 3*), and, finally, "On the whole, the text does not read fluently" (*below TDN 3*). The descriptor-specific TDNs were aggregated to yield a single TDN rating for each criterion.

Taken together, there were 648 ratings on each criterion; that is, 614 double ratings plus 34 third ratings, making a total of 1,944 ratings. These ratings provided the input for estimating parameters based on the MFRM model specified in the next section.

For illustrative purposes, Table 2.1 presents an excerpt from the essay rating data. Each line in the table shows which examinee received which scores from which rater on each criterion. For example, Examinee 001 was rated by Rater 01; this examinee received *TDN 5* on both *global impression* (GI) and *task fulfillment* (TF), and *TDN 4* on *linguistic realization* (LR). Note that Examinee 131 was additionally rated by a third rater (i.e., Rater 06). As mentioned above, this rater provided the necessary link between examinees, raters, and criteria.

2.2.3 Rasch modeling of essay rating data

The preceding description of the essay rating data suggests that there were three relevant facets: examinees, raters, and criteria. In terms of the MFRM approach, any element of the examinee facet combines with any element of the rater facet and with any element of the criterion facet to produce an observation (rating, score) on the four-category rating scale.

Assuming a constant structure of the rating scale across the elements of each of the three facets, the basic MFRM model suitable for an analysis of the essay-rating data can be specified as follows:

$$\ln\left[\frac{p_{nijk}}{p_{nijk-1}}\right] = \theta_n - \beta_i - \alpha_j - \tau_k, \qquad (2.11)$$

where

p_{nijk}	=	probability of examinee *n* receiving a rating of *k* from rater *j* on criterion *i*,
p_{nijk-1}	=	probability of examinee *n* receiving a rating of *k* – 1 from rater *j* on criterion *i*,
θ_n	=	ability of examinee *n*,
β_i	=	difficulty of criterion *i*,
α_j	=	severity of rater *j*,
τ_k	=	difficulty of receiving a rating of *k* relative to *k* – 1.

Results from the MFRM analysis based on the model shown in Equation 2.11 will be presented in detail later, particularly in Chapters 4 through 7. Chapter 4 provides a first look at the joint calibration of examinees, raters, and criteria. In Chapter 5, the focus is on rater measurement results, including a discussion of rater fit statistics. When dealing with examinee measurement results in Chapter 6, the attention shifts to the issue of ensuring fairness in performance assessments. Chapter 7 provides detail on the criterion measures and probes into the structure and the effectiveness of the rating scale.

First though, in the next chapter, some basic issues revolving around rater-mediated assessment will be discussed. Chapter 3 elaborates on the error-proneness of human ratings, the serious limitations of traditional approaches to addressing rating error, and the complexity of the rating task facing human raters. In so doing, the chapter lays the groundwork for answering the question of why it is fundamentally important to go beyond the raw scores typically provided in performance assessments.

3. Rater-Mediated Assessment: Meeting the Challenge

Human raters are fallible: Each time a rater provides a score that is meant to express an evaluation of the quality of an examinee's response to a particular task, that score is likely to misrepresent the proficiency of the examinee to some extent. However, raters are not the only source of measurement error. A host of other facets also come into play that may have a similarly adverse impact on the assessment outcomes. This chapter first discusses the notorious problem of rater variability and presents the standard approach to dealing with that problem. Then the essay rating data are used to illustrate the computation and interpretation of different indices of interrater reliability and to highlight the limitations of the standard approach. The final section outlines the conceptual–psychometric framework that underlies the Rasch measurement approach to meeting the challenge of rater-mediated assessment.

3.1 Rater variability

Performance assessments typically employ constructed-response items, requiring examinees to create a response, rather than choose the correct answer from alternatives given. To arrive at scores capturing the intended proficiency, raters have to closely attend to, interpret, and evaluate the responses that examinees provide. In keeping with the rater cognition perspective of performance assessment (e.g., Bejar, 2012; Lumley, 2005; see also Section 10.4), the process of assessing examinee performance can be described as a complex and indirect one: Examinees respond to assessment items or tasks designed to represent the underlying construct, and raters perceive, interpret, and evaluate the responses building on their understanding of that construct and on their understanding of the scoring guidelines or rubrics (Bejar, Williamson, & Mislevy, 2006; Freedman & Calfee, 1983; Lumley, 2005; McNamara, 1996; Wolfe, 1997). This long, and possibly fragile, interpretation–evaluation–scoring chain highlights the need to carefully investigate the psychometric quality of rater-mediated assessments. One of the major difficulties facing the researcher, and the practitioner alike, is the occurrence of rater variability.

The term *rater variability* generally refers to variability of scores awarded to examinees that is associated with characteristics of the raters and not with the performance of examinees. Put differently, rater variability is a component of unwanted variability contributing to *construct-irrelevant variance* in performance assessments (Haladyna & Downing, 2004; Messick, 1989, 1995). This kind of variability obscures the construct being measured and, therefore, threatens the validity and fairness of assessment outcomes, their interpretation, and use (Lane & Stone, 2006; McNamara & Roever, 2006; Weir, 2005). Related terms like *rater effects* (Houston, Raymond, & Svec, 1991; Myford & Wolfe, 2003, 2004), *rater error* (Downing, 2005; Saal et al., 1980), or *rater bias* (Hoyt, 2000; Johnson et al., 2009), each touch on the fundamental rater variability problem.

Common rater effects, besides the severity effect discussed earlier, are halo and central tendency effects. A *central tendency effect* is exhibited when raters avoid the extreme categories of a rating scale and prefer categories near the scale midpoint instead. Ratings based on an analytic scoring rubric may be susceptible to a *halo effect*. This effect manifests itself when raters fail to distinguish between conceptually distinct scoring criteria, providing excessively similar ratings across these criteria; for example, ratings may be influenced by an overall impression of a given performance or dominated by a single feature viewed as highly important. In a MFRM framework, central tendency and halo effects can be examined indirectly (e.g., Engelhard, 2002; Knoch, 2009a; Linacre, 2014b; Myford & Wolfe, 2003, 2004; Wolfe, 2004). Statistical indicators that may be used to detect each of these effects are dealt with in Chapter 5.

Obviously, then, rater variability is not a unitary phenomenon, but can manifest itself in various forms that each call for close scrutiny. Research has shown that raters may differ not only in the degree of severity or leniency exhibited when scoring examinee performance, but also in the degree to which they comply with the scoring rubric, in the way they interpret scoring criteria, in their understanding and use of rating scale categories, or in the degree to which their ratings are consistent across examinees, scoring criteria, performance tasks, assessment time, and other facets involved (see Bachman and Palmer, 1996; Brown, 2005; Hamp-Lyons, 2007; Lumley, 2005; McNamara, 1996; Weigle, 2002).

The usual, or standard, approach to come to grips with rater variability, especially in high-stakes assessments, consists of three components: rater training, independent ratings of the same performance by two or more raters (repeated ratings), and establishing interrater reliability. The first component, *rater training*, typically pursues the goal of familiarizing raters with the format of the assessment, the tasks, and the rating procedure (Johnson et al., 2009; Lane & Stone, 2006; Van Moere, 2014; Xi & Mollaun, 2009). More specifically, raters are trained with the aim to achieve a common understanding of (a) the construct being measured, (b) the level, or levels, of performance the assessment is aiming at, (c) the criteria and the associated descriptors that represent the construct at each performance level, (d) the categories of the rating scale or scales, and (e) the overall difficulty level of the items or tasks to which examinees are to respond.

A time-honored safeguard against the occurrence of rater effects is the use of *repeated* or *multiple ratings* of the same performance. However, such ratings typically reveal considerable disagreement among raters. In these cases, those who supervise the raters must decide how to handle the disagreements in order to arrive at a final score for an examinee. The literature is replete with different disagreement resolution procedures, including averaging the complete set of independent ratings, using only those ratings that are in sufficiently close agreement, or calling in an expert rater (e.g., Johnson et al., 2009; Myford & Wolfe, 2002).

Ideally, differences between raters that may exist after training should be practically unimportant; that is, *interrater reliability* should be close to its maximum value possible. Yet, research has shown that this ideal is extremely difficult to achieve in most situations. Raters typically remain far from functioning interchangeably even after extensive training sessions (Barrett, 2001; Eckes, 2004, 2005b, 2010a; Elbow & Yancey, 1994; Houston & Myford, 2009; Hoyt & Kerns, 1999; Kondo-Brown, 2002; Lumley & McNamara, 1995; O'Sullivan & Rignall, 2007; Weigle, 1998, 1999; Yan, 2014). Moreover, the provision of detailed individualized feedback to raters does not seem to remedy the problem (Elder, Knoch, Barkhuizen, & von Randow, 2005; Elder, Barkhuizen, Knoch, & von Randow, 2007; Knoch, Read, & von Randow, 2007). For example, Knoch (2011) investigated the effectiveness of providing detailed feedback to raters longitudinally, after each of four assessment administrations. She concluded that "ratings were no better (in terms of severity, bias and consistency) when raters were given feedback than when they were not" (p. 199).

Moreover, trained, experienced raters have been shown to differ systematically in their interpretation of scoring criteria. Rather than forming a single, homogeneous group having a common understanding of how to interpret and use criteria, raters appear to fall into *rater types*, with each type characterized by a distinct scoring focus, decision-making strategy, or rating style (e.g., Crisp, 2008; Cumming, 1990; Eckes, 2008b; Gamaroff, 2000; Shaw, 2007). In language assessment, for example, some raters manifested a strong focus on criteria referring to vocabulary and syntax, whereas others put significantly more weight on structure or fluency (Eckes, 2008b, 2009b). Rater types were also associated with criterion-related biases in operational writing assessment contexts, with more severe ratings on criteria perceived as highly important (Eckes, 2012; He, Gou, Chien, Chen, & Chang, 2013; see also Section 10.4).

3.2 Interrater reliability

3.2.1 The standard approach

As explained above, the trilogy of rater training, repeated ratings, and demonstration of interrater reliability is the hallmark of the standard approach to addressing the rater variability problem. The usual assumption is this: If interrater reliability is sufficiently high, then raters share the same view of the construct and also the same view of the rating scale; as a result, they will provide accurate ratings in terms of coming close to an examinee's "true" level of proficiency. However, this assumption is flawed.

To begin with, even if high interrater reliability has been achieved in a given assessment context, exactly what such a finding stands for may be far from clear. One reason for this is that there is no commonly accepted definition of interrater reliability. Over time, interrater reliability has come to be conceptualized in many different ways, by many different people, and for many different purposes, resulting in a bewildering array of indices (e.g., Bramley, 2007; Cherry & Meyer, 1993; Hayes & Krippendorff, 2007; LeBreton & Senter, 2008; Morgan, Zhu, Johnson, & Hodge, 2014; Schuster & Smith, 2005; Shoukri, 2004; von Eye & Mun, 2005; Zegers, 1991). To complicate matters, different coefficients of interrater reliability can mean vastly different things.

In this situation, it seems helpful to distinguish between two broad classes of indices: consensus indices and consistency indices (Stemler & Tsai, 2008; Tinsley & Weiss, 1975, 2000). Specifically, a *consensus index* of interrater reliability, also called *interrater agreement*, refers to the extent to which independent raters provide the same rating of a particular examinee or object (absolute correspondence of ratings). In contrast, a *consistency index* of interrater reliability refers to the extent to which independent raters provide the same relative ordering or ranking of the examinees or objects being rated (relative correspondence of ratings).

Though often used interchangeably in the literature, indices from these two classes can lead to discrepant, sometimes even contradictory results and conclusions. It is possible to observe low interrater consensus and, at the same time, high interrater consistency (and vice versa). For example, one rater may award scores to examinees that are consistently one or two scale points lower than the scores that another rater awards to the same examinees. The relative ordering of the examinees will be much the same for both raters, yielding high consistency estimates; yet, the raters have *not* reached exact agreement in any one case.

In the next two sections, I discuss in more detail the distinction between consensus and consistency indices, as well as serious limitations of these classes of indices, building on the essay rating data described previously. Note that there are indices of interrater reliability that belong to both classes. For example, some variants of the intraclass correlation coefficient are a function of both rater consensus and rater consistency (e.g., LeBreton & Senter, 2008; McGraw & Wong, 1996).

3.2.2 Consensus and consistency

In order to compute indices of interrater reliability, a single TDN level representing each rater's total evaluation of a given essay was derived as follows. First, the individual criterion-related ratings that each rater awarded to an essay were averaged across the three criteria, that is, across the ratings on *global impression*, *task fulfillment*, and *linguistic realization*. Then, the obtained averages were rounded to the next TDN level.[2]

Based on the final, aggregate TDN levels, two commonly used indices of consensus and consistency, respectively, were computed. The resulting consensus and consistency values serve to highlight the critical difference between both classes of reliability indices.

Table 3.1: Consensus and Consistency Indices of Interrater Reliability (Sample Data).

		Consensus Indices		Consistency Indices	
Rater Pair	***N***	**Exact Agreement**	**Cohen's Weighted Kappa**	**Pearson's *r***	**Kendall's Tau-b**
07 / 10	20	.70	.67	.83	.78
13 / 16	20	.60	.67	.84	.84
12 / 03	20	.55	.29	.49	.42

2 The rounding rule used here was as follows: average scores smaller than 2.50 were assigned to level *below TDN 3*, average scores from 2.50 to 3.49 to *TDN 3*, average scores from 3.50 to 4.49 to *TDN 4*, and average scores greater than 4.49 to *TDN 5*. For the purposes of computation, *below TDN 3* was scored "2", the other levels were scored from "3" to "5".

		Consensus Indices		Consistency Indices	
Rater Pair	*N*	Exact Agreement	Cohen's Weighted Kappa	Pearson's *r*	Kendall's Tau-b
17 / 11	19	.53	.42	.62	.58
14 / 08	23	.52	.50	.77	.70
08 / 12	24	.50	.54	.71	.64
09 / 17	26	.50	.34	.53	.49
05 / 18	21	.48	.53	.76	.68
02 / 04	24	.46	.33	.58	.52
10 / 09	21	.43	.41	.78	.72
15 / 07	28	.36	.20	.53	.48
13 / 03	21	.24	.22	.66	.62
05 / 07	20	.20	.22	.77	.72
01 / 14	20	.10	.00	.21	.26

Note. Each essay was independently rated by two raters on a four-category rating scale. N = number of essays rated by a given pair of raters.

Consensus indices were the *exact agreement index* and *Cohen's weighted kappa*. Exact agreement was defined as the number of essays that received identical ratings, divided by the total number of essays rated by the two raters. The kappa index corrects the agreement between raters for agreement expected on the basis of chance alone. Since the four TDN levels were ordered, the weighted version of kappa (Cohen, 1968) based on a linear weighting scheme was used; that is, successively less weight was assigned to disagreement when categories were farther apart (weights of 0.67, 0.33, and 0.0 for differences of 1, 2, or 3 categories, respectively). Weighted kappa has a maximum of 1 when agreement is perfect, a value of 0 indicates no agreement better than chance, and negative values show worse than chance agreement (e.g., Fleiss, Levin, & Paik, 2003; Mun, 2005).

Consistency indices were the *product–moment correlation* and *Kendall's tau-b*. The product–moment correlation coefficient (also called Pearson's *r*) reflects the degree of linear relationship between the ratings of two raters. Kendall's tau-b reflects the degree of correspondence between two rank orderings of examinee performances, taking tied ranks into account. Both reliability indices range from 0 to 1, with higher values indicating a stronger correlation or correspondence between ratings.

Table 3.1 gives the consensus and consistency results for 14 pairs of raters. The rater pairs are ordered from high to low exact agreement. All raters listed in the table belonged to the panel of 17 operational raters involved in rating examinee performance. As mentioned previously, there was one rater (i.e., Rater 06) whose ratings solely served to satisfy the connectedness requirement. Therefore, this rater was not included in the table. The number of common ratings per rater pair varied between 19 essays (rater pair 17/11) and 28 essays (rater pair 15/07).

Exact agreement ranged from an acceptably high value of .70 for Raters 07 and 10 to a strikingly low value of .10 for Raters 01 and 14. Most agreement values were in the .40s and .50s, much too low to be satisfactory within a high-stakes context (Fleiss et al., 2003); weighted kappa reached values that could be judged as sufficiently high only for two pairs (i.e., rater pairs 07/10 and 13/16). In one case, the agreement rate was exactly at a level predicted by chance alone (rater pair 01/14).

Consensus and consistency indices suggested much the same conclusions for the majority of rater pairs. There were two notable exceptions, however. These exceptions concerned Raters 13 and 03, and Raters 05 and 07, respectively. For these two rater pairs, consistency values were moderately high, but consensus values turned out to be much too low to be considered acceptable.

3.2.3 Limitations of the standard approach

To gain more insight into the problems associated with the standard approach, first look at rater pair 13/16. For these two raters, fairly good consensus and consistency values were obtained. Table 3.2 presents the cross-classification of the observed rating frequencies.[3]

Raters 13 and 16 arrived at identical ratings in 12 cases (shown in the shaded cells), they disagreed in eight cases. Each disagreement concerned only one TDN level. For example, four examinees received *TDN 4* by Rater 13, but *TDN 3* by Rater 16.

Now look at Rater 13 again, but this time in relation to Rater 03 (see Table 3.3).

There were 16 cases of disagreement, 10 of which concerned one TDN level, and the remaining six cases each concerned two TDN levels. For example,

3 In the CEFR Manual (Council of Europe, 2009), tables like these are called "bivariate decision tables".

four examinees received *TDN 3* by Rater 13, but *TDN 5* by Rater 03. However, the disagreements appeared to be anything but random. There was not a single case in which Rater 03 provided a lower rating than Rater 13. Thus, Rater 03 exhibited a tendency to award *systematically higher* levels than Rater 13.

The pattern of disagreements for pair 13/03 suggests the following tentative conclusion: Rater 13 disagreed with Rater 03 so strongly because he or she was more *severe* than Rater 03, or, conversely, because Rater 03 was more *lenient* than Rater 13.

Table 3.2: Cross-Classification of Rating Frequencies for Raters 13 and 16.

	Rater 16				
Rater 13	**b. TDN 3**	**TDN 3**	**TDN 4**	**TDN 5**	**Row total**
below TDN 3	**8**				8
TDN 3	**1**	**1**			2
TDN 4		**4**	**2**	**3**	9
TDN 5				**1**	1
Column total	9	5	2	4	20

Note. Consensus indices are .60 (exact agreement) and .67 (Cohen's weighted kappa). Consistency indices are .84 (Pearson's *r*) and .84 (Kendall's tau-b).

Table 3.3: Cross-Classification of Rating Frequencies for Raters 13 and 03.

	Rater 03				
Rater 13	**b. TDN 3**	**TDN 3**	**TDN 4**	**TDN 5**	**Row total**
below TDN 3	**1**	**3**	**2**		6
TDN 3			**5**	**4**	9
TDN 4			**2**	**2**	4
TDN 5				**2**	2
Column total	1	3	9	8	21

Note. Consensus indices are .24 (exact agreement) and .22 (Cohen's weighted kappa). Consistency indices are .66 (Pearson's *r*) and .62 (Kendall's tau-b).

This difference in severity or leniency, respectively, could account for the fact that consensus indices were unacceptably low, whereas consistency indices were considerably higher. As explained previously, consistency indices of interrater reliability are sensitive to the relative ordering of examinees. These orderings of examinees, as evident in each of the raters' final ratings, were indeed highly congruent.

Given that this conclusion is correct: what about the high reliability indices (in terms of both consensus and consistency) observed for Raters 13 and 16? Could it not be that these two raters were characterized by much the same degree of severity or leniency, respectively, and that on these grounds they provided highly similar ratings in the majority of cases? And, when similar degrees of severity/leniency accounted for satisfactorily high consensus and consistency observed for these two raters, would it be reasonable to call their ratings "accurate"?

These questions point to a fundamental problem of the standard approach to interrater reliability, a problem that may be dubbed the *agreement–accuracy paradox*. High consensus or agreement among raters, and in this sense, high reliability, does not necessarily imply high accuracy in assessing examinee proficiency. Neither does high consistency imply high accuracy, even if consensus is high. Thus, high reliability may lead to the wrong conclusion that raters provided highly accurate ratings when in fact they did not (see also Henning, 1996).

What about raters exhibiting low consensus *and* low consistency? One could be tempted to consider their ratings as misleading, and to dismiss these raters or replace them by more reliable raters. For example, Tinsley and Weiss (2000, p. 101) arrived at the conclusion that, when both consensus and consistency are low, "the ratings have no validity and should not be used for research or applied purposes". Let us have a look at a final example illustrating that this conclusion is not appropriate.

Table 3.4 presents the cross-classification of rating frequencies for Raters 01 and 14. Of all raters considered in the present sample, these two raters had the lowest consensus and consistency values. They agreed exactly in only two out of 20 cases, and this agreement rate could be accounted for by chance alone. However, the distribution of rating frequencies still showed some regularity. Specifically, both raters used a restricted range of the TDN scale: Rater 14 only used scale categories *TDN 3* to *TDN 5*, and Rater 01 only used scale categories *TDN 4* and *TDN 5*. Moreover, Rater 01 awarded higher scores in 17 cases (i.e., 85%), suggesting a clear tendency to be more lenient than Rater 14. Obviously, then, this kind of regularity is missed when the standard approach is adopted.

Table 3.4: Cross-Classification of Rating Frequencies for Raters 01 and 14.

	Rater 14				
Rater 01	**b. TDN 3**	**TDN 3**	**TDN 4**	**TDN 5**	**Row total**
below TDN 3					0
TDN 3					0
TDN 4		**6**	**1**	**1**	8
TDN 5		**5**	**6**	**1**	12
Column total	0	11	7	2	20

Note. Consensus indices are .10 (exact agreement) and .00 (Cohen's weighted kappa). Consistency indices are .21 (Pearson's *r*) and .26 (Kendall's tau-b).

Falling back on alternative consensus or consistency indices of interrater reliability is no way out of the fundamental dilemma. The difficulties in adequately representing the structure inherent in the rating data will remain as long as the underlying rationale is the same. The paradox exemplified here can only be resolved when the standard approach is abandoned in favor of a measurement approach.

Basically, many-facet Rasch measurement yields an in-depth account of the similarities and differences in raters' views when assessing examinees' proficiency. Later I will show how the sample data can be analyzed using a MFRM approach. First, though, I want to broaden the perspective and go into somewhat more detail regarding the various sources of variability in ratings that are typical of rater-mediated assessments.

3.3 A conceptual-psychometric framework

The MFRM sample data analysis rests on a conceptual model of facets that potentially influence the assessment of examinee writing performance. Figure 3.1 depicts these facets, highlights some of their mutual relationships, and relates them to typical MFRM output.[4]

To be sure, the facets shown do not encompass all that may happen in a particular assessment context. The rating process is undoubtedly far more complex and dynamic than can be summarized in a diagram, and the facets coming into play are diverse at any given moment (e.g., Engelhard, 2013; Engelhard & Myford, 2003; Lane & Stone, 2006; McNamara, 1995, 1996; Murphy & Cleveland, 1995; Shaw, 2007).

4 Figure 3.1 is an extended version of a figure presented earlier (see, e.g., Eckes, 2005a, 2008a, 2010a).

Fig. 3.1: A conceptual–psychometric framework of rater-mediated assessment.

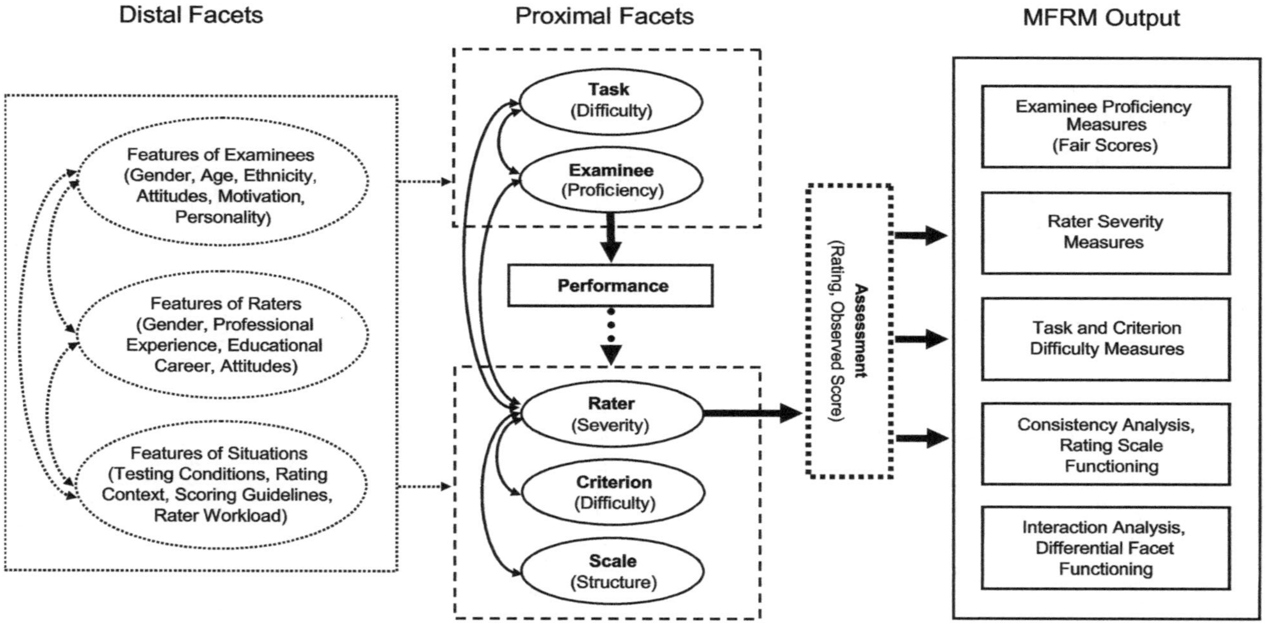

Each facet, and each facet interrelation, that is identified in an assessment constitutes a potential source of variation in the ratings. Assumptions about relevant facets may originate from previous research on the subject matter, from observations made in similar assessment contexts, or from earlier modeling attempts that turned out to be unsatisfactory. For example, in the early stages of the measurement process it may happen that some relevant facets go unnoticed; these facets are called *hidden facets*. The presence of hidden facets can have deleterious effects on the measurement results, such as yielding biased estimates of examinee proficiency.

Note also that the diagram refers to facets usually involved in *writing* performance assessments. Assessing *speaking* performance is often more intricate still, particularly in direct speaking assessments (Berry, 2007; Brown, 2005; Eckes, 2010b; Fulcher, 2003; Galaczi, 2010; O'Loughlin, 2001; O'Sullivan, 2008). For example, when speaking proficiency is assessed through face-to-face interaction, facets that may additionally affect examinee performance often relate to interviewers, interlocutors, and other examinees being simultaneously present in the assessment (Bachman, 2002; Davis, 2009; Ockey, 2009; Van Moere, 2006).

With these caveats in mind, the following outline will help to prepare the stage for introducing more specific concepts relevant for a detailed psychometric analysis of performance assessments.

3.3.1 Proximal and distal facets

Consider first the facets shown in the middle part of Figure 3.1. This part comprises facets that have an immediate impact on the scores awarded to examinees. In the following, these facets are called *proximal* facets. The single most important proximal facet is the proficiency of an examinee representing the construct to be measured (e.g., writing proficiency). To highlight the prominent role of examinee proficiency in the assessment process, this facet is shown in an ellipse with an unbroken line. The same graphic symbol is used to designate the other proximal facets.

One of these other facets refers to the difficulty of the task, or tasks, examinees are asked to respond to. Note that the very same task may be relatively easy for one group of examinees and relatively difficult for another group for reasons that need not readily be known; for example, examinees may differ to some extent in the background knowledge brought to bear on a particular task. Put another way, examinees and tasks may *interact* with one another. This kind of interaction, represented in the figure through a two-way arrow linking examinee and task, may by itself have an impact on examinee performance. Alternatively, when examinees are free to choose from among a given number of tasks differing in difficulty, the choice of a difficult task is likely to result in a lower performance than the choice of a less difficult task. The net effect would be an increase in the variability of examinee scores not attributable to underlying proficiency, that is, an increase in construct-irrelevant variance.

Other proximal facets that are basically irrelevant to the construct and thus potentially contribute to systematic measurement error in the ratings are shown in the lower section of the middle part. These include rater severity and scoring criterion difficulty, discussed in depth later. Finally, a less obvious source of measurement error concerns variability in the structure of the rating scale, or scales, used. That is, the ordered categories of a given rating scale may change their meaning between raters, within raters over time, between tasks or between criteria (Knoch, 2009b; Weigle, 2002). For example, raters may differ from each other in their interpretation of the ordering of scale categories; that is, some raters may actually perceive two adjacent categories, or the performance levels implied by these categories, to be much closer together than other raters do.

For ease of presentation, Figure 3.1 only includes two-way interactions. In some instances, however, three-way or even higher-way interactions between proximal facets may come into play. As an example of a three-way interaction consider the case that some raters tended to award unexpectedly low scores on scoring criteria referring to task fulfillment when rating low-proficiency examinees, and unexpectedly high scores on scoring criteria referring to linguistic realization when rating high-proficiency examinees.

Moreover, to illustrate that the route from examinee performance to an observed score (rating, raw score) is typically long and fragile, as discussed in the beginning of the chapter, the link from performance to the set of rater-related proximal facets is represented by a dotted arrow. That is, the score a rater awards to an examinee is the result of a complex interplay between bottom-up, performance-driven processes (e.g., distinct features of the performance) and top-down, theory-driven (knowledge-driven) processes (e.g., expectations based on knowledge of prior examinee performance or based on gender, age, ethnic, or other social categories). Viewed from the perspective of rater cognition research, an important role is to be assigned to performance features as perceived by raters, and to the features' mapping to the criteria and the rating scale categories as usually spelled out in the scoring rubrics (Eckes, 2008b, 2012; Lumley, 2005; Wolfe, 1997).

The left-hand side of Figure 3.1 shows three categories of variables that may exert additional influence on the ratings, albeit usually in a more indirect, mediated, or diffuse way. These variables are called *distal* facets. In the figure, each of these is illustrated by an ellipse with a dotted line. Distal facets refer to (a) features of examinees (e.g., gender, ethnicity, first language, personality traits, beliefs, goals), (b) features of raters (e.g., number of foreign languages spoken, professional background, educational career, goals, and motivation), and (c) features of situations, that is, features of the assessment or rating context (e.g., physical environment, rater workload, time of rating, paper-based vs. onscreen scoring, quality management policy). Some of the distal facets may interact with one another and may also interact with some of the proximal facets, such as when examinee gender interacts with rater severity or when raters' degree of professional experience interacts with their interpretation of scoring criteria.

3.3.2 A measurement approach

Adopting a measurement approach to dealing with the challenge of rater-mediated assessment allows the researcher to gain a fine-grained view of the functioning of the assessment system employed. To illustrate, the right-hand side of Figure 3.1 shows major types of output from a MFRM analysis. Thus, MFRM modeling generally provides a well-structured and detailed account of the role played by each facet (proximal and/or distal) that is deemed relevant in a given assessment context. In the following, basic concepts are introduced in a non-technical manner just to give a first impression of the range of available procedures. More detail, including the specification of an appropriate MFRM model and formal definitions of statistical indicators, is provided in subsequent chapters.

As discussed in Chapter 2, the MFRM model is an extension of the basic Rasch model. This extension is twofold: (a) there is no restriction to the analysis of only two facets (i.e., examinees and items), and (b) the data being analyzed need not be dichotomous. In an analysis of performance assessments, the MFRM model allows one to take account of additional facets of that setting that may be of particular interest, such as raters, tasks, and criteria. Moreover, raters typically award scores to examinees using ordered scale categories (i.e., rating scales). Therefore, the data in most instances comprise polytomous responses.

Within each facet, the model represents each element (i.e., each individual examinee, rater, task, criterion, etc.) by a separate parameter value. The parameters denote distinct attributes of the facets involved, such as proficiency (for examinees), severity (for raters), and difficulty (for items, tasks, or scoring criteria). In many assessment contexts, the measure of primary interest refers to examinees. Specifically, for each examinee, a MFRM analysis provides a proficiency measure (in logits). Following the principle of measurement invariance, when the data fit the model, these measures compensate for between-rater severity; that is, the examinee proficiency measures are adjusted for differences in the levels of severity of the raters who assigned the ratings. In addition, the analysis yields a standard error that indicates the precision of each proficiency measure.

On the basis of MFRM model parameter estimates, a *fair score* (fair average, expected score) can be derived for each examinee (Linacre, 2014b). Fair scores result from a transformation of examinee proficiency estimates reported in logits to the corresponding scores on the raw-score scale. That is, a fair score is the score that a particular examinee would have obtained from a rater of average severity. Fair scores thus illustrate the effect of the model-based compensation for between-rater severity/leniency differences.

When a MFRM analysis is run, the specified facets are analyzed simultaneously and calibrated onto a single linear scale (i.e., the logit scale). The joint calibration of facets makes it possible to measure rater severity on the same scale as examinee proficiency, task difficulty, and criterion difficulty. By placing all parameter estimates on a common scale, a frame of reference for interpreting the results is constructed. Therefore, if the data show sufficient fit to the model, measures of examinee proficiency, rater severity, task difficulty, and criterion difficulty can be directly compared to each other.

A MFRM analysis provides, for each element of each facet, *fit indices* showing the degree to which observed ratings match the expected ratings that are generated by the model. Regarding the rater facet, fit indices provide estimates of the consistency with which each individual rater made use of the scale categories across examinees, tasks, and criteria. A *consistency analysis* based on the inspection of rater fit indices has an important role to play in rater monitoring and rater training, especially when it comes to providing feedback to raters on their rating behavior. Fit indices may also help to detect various rater effects besides severity/leniency, such as central tendency or halo effects (Engelhard, 2002; Knoch et al., 2007; Myford & Wolfe, 2003, 2004; Wolfe, 2004; Wolfe & McVay, 2012).

In performance assessments, the input data to a MFRM analysis generally are ratings based on a set, or sets, of ordered response categories. How well these categories, that is, the scores awarded to examinees, are separated from one another is an empirical question directly relevant to establishing the psychometric quality of the data. A MFRM analysis typically provides a number of useful indices for studying the functioning of rating scales. For example, for each rating scale category, the average of the examinee proficiency measures that went into the calculation of the category measure should advance monotonically with categories. When this pattern is borne out in the data, the results suggest that examinees with higher ratings are indeed exhibiting "more" of the variable that is being measured than examinees with lower ratings.

Once the parameters of a MFRM model have been estimated, possible interaction effects, such as the interaction between raters and examinees or between examinees and tasks, can be investigated. To this end, the basic MFRM model needs to be extended to include interaction terms that represent the deviation of particular combinations of between-facet elements (e.g., rater–examinee pairs) from their average parameter estimates (raters and examinees, respectively).

An *interaction analysis* helps to identify unusual patterns of observations among various facet elements, particularly those patterns that suggest consistent deviations from what is expected on the basis of the model. The occurrence of such deviations would indicate the presence of *differential facet functioning* (Du, Wright, & Brown, 1996; Engelhard, 2002; Wang, 2000).

4. Many-Facet Rasch Analysis: A First Look

In this chapter, the basic MFRM modeling approach is explained using the essay rating data. First, various steps that need to be taken in preparation for a MFRM analysis are discussed. This includes formatting the input data and building a specification file. A key component of the results is a graphical display showing the joint calibration of examinees, raters, criteria, and the rating scale categories. Each part of this display is explained with respect to its substantive implications. Then, statistical indicators that summarize information on the variability within each facet are formally described and, in a subsequent section, applied to the sample data. The focus is on the different meanings these indicators may assume depending on the facet under consideration. The chapter concludes with a brief look at the contentious issue of global model fit.

4.1 Preparing for a many-facet Rasch analysis

To summarize briefly, the input data consisted of ratings that 18 raters awarded to essays written by 307 examinees in a live examination. Each essay was independently rated by at least two raters according to three criteria. Ratings were provided along the four-category TDN scale (with TDN levels scored from 2 to 5).

The data were analyzed by means of the computer program FACETS (Version 3.71; Linacre, 2014a). This program used the scores that raters awarded to examinees to estimate individual examinee proficiencies, rater severities, criterion difficulties, and scale category difficulties. FACETS accepts data files, with their data correctly formatted, coming from various sources, such as Excel, R, SAS, SPSS, or STATA; in addition, FACETS is accompanied by a separate data formatting program called FACFORM (Linacre, 2009), which can be used for building FACETS data files.

Besides an input data file, FACETS requires a specification file that contains the instructions on how to analyze the data. Table 4.1 presents an excerpt from the specification file used for the present sample data analysis.

The left column of Table 4.1 lists control variables and commands; explanations are provided in the right column. Most importantly, the command "Model=?,?,?,R5" defines the model to be used in the analysis—the three-facet rating scale model (RSM) as shown in Equation 2.11 (Section 2.2.3). If one wanted instead to perform a partial-credit analysis where each rater is modeled separately to take into account his or her own use of the rating scale, the model definition would look like this: "Model=?,#,?,R5"; that is, the symbol "#" would specify a PCM for the individual elements of the rater facet (see also Section 8.3).

In order to establish the origin of the logit scale and to make the model identifiable, the rater and criterion facets are centered; that is, these facets are constrained to have a mean element measure of zero. Similarly, the sum of the category coefficients is required to equal zero (this is a default not listed in the specification file). Hence, as in most cases, the examinee facet is the only facet left non-centered ("Noncenter = 1"). The next command, "Positive=1", says that only the first facet (i.e., the examinee facet) is to be measured positively; that is, a high proficiency measure means the raw score is high, and a low proficiency measure means the raw score is low. At the same time, raters are to be measured negatively, such that higher severity measures indicate lower scores awarded to examinees (the default option in educational measurement). This also applies to the criterion facet; that is, higher difficulty measures indicate lower scores. If, for some reason or other, measurement results were to be communicated in terms of rater leniency and criterion easiness, these two facets would be included in the command; that is, "Positive=1,2,3" would define all three facets as positively oriented.

The graphical display of the measurement results is specified by the control variable "Vertical=". With this variable, as with most of the other variables, FACETS users have many options available to tailor the graphical output to their needs. For example, when the vertical rulers were to show raters by number (i.e., the entry number in the data file) instead of raters by label, the command would be "Vertical=1*,2N,3A". The next section discusses the vertical rulers as defined by the command given in Table 4.1.

Table 4.1: Excerpt from the FACETS Specification File for the Sample Data Analysis (Control Variables, Commands, and Explanations).

Specification	Explanation
Title = Essay rating	Title of the MFRM analysis.
Facets = 3	There are three facets involved in producing the observations: examinees, raters, criteria.
Data file = W002.txt	The input data are in a separate file.

Specification	Explanation
Model = ?,?,?,R5	Model definition: any examinee ("?") can combine with any rater ("?") and with any criterion ("?") to produce a rating (R); R5 indicates the highest category of the rating scale (i.e., 5); the four-category rating scale is assumed to function in a similar manner across all raters and all criteria (RSM).
*	End of model definition.
Noncenter = 1	Except Facet 1 (examinees), elements of all facets are centered. This establishes the origin of the measurement scale.
Positive = 1	For Facet 1 (examinees), higher measure means higher score; for the remaining facets (raters, criteria), higher measure means lower score.
Inter-rater = 2	Agreement statistics are computed for Facet 2 (raters).
Vertical = 1*,2A,3A	The variable map shows examinees by distribution ("*"); raters and criteria are shown by label ("A").
Labels =	The list of labels (identifiers) follows:
1,Examinee	Facet 1, the examinee facet.
1=001	001 is the label of the first examinee.
…	(Examinees 002 to 306 to follow here.)
307=307	307 is the label of the last examinee.
*	End of Facet 1.
2,Rater	Facet 2, the rater facet.
1=01	01 is the label of the first rater.
…	(Raters 02 to 17 to follow here.)
18=18	18 is the label of the last rater.
*	End of Facet 2.
3,Criterion	Facet 3, the criterion facet.
1=GI	GI is the label of the first criterion, global impression.
2=TF	TF is the label of the second criterion, task fulfillment.
3=LR	LR is the label of the third criterion, linguistic realization.
*	End of Facet 3.

4.2 Measures at a glance: The Wright map

The FACETS program calibrated the examinees, raters, and criteria, as well as the rating scale onto the logit scale, creating a single frame of reference for interpreting the results of the analysis. Representing these calibrations, Figure 4.1 displays the *Wright map*, or *variable map*. This map, named after Benjamin D. Wright (see Wilson, 2005, 2011), is a highly informative piece of output, showing the *vertical rulers* and thus facilitating direct comparisons between, and within, the facets under consideration.

In the Wright map, the measurement scale appears as the first column (labeled "Logit"). In the same basic way that examinee ability and item difficulty were located on the same (horizontal) dimension in the two-facet dichotomous case (see Figure 2.1), all measures of examinees, raters, and criteria, as well as the category coefficients, are now positioned vertically on the same latent dimension, with logits as measurement units.

The second column ("Examinees") displays the estimates of the examinee proficiency parameter. Here, each star represents three examinees, and a dot represents one or two examinees (for illustrative purposes). Proficiency measures are ordered with higher-scoring examinees appearing at the top of the column, and lower-scoring examinees appearing at the bottom. Thus, the examinee facet is positively oriented, as previously defined in the specification file (see Table 4.1).[5]

The third column ("Raters") compares the raters in terms of the level of severity each exercised when rating essays. More severe raters appear higher in the column, while less severe (or more lenient) raters appear lower; that is, the rater facet has a negative orientation. As mentioned earlier, the basic measurement model could also be defined in terms of rater leniency. Then, in Equation 2.11, the rater term would be added instead of being subtracted, and the elements in the rater column (Figure 4.1) would be in reverse order, with more lenient raters at the top of the column, and more severe raters at the bottom.

As can be seen, the variability across raters in their level of severity was substantial. In fact, the rater severity measures showed a 4.64-logit spread, which was about a third (31.1%) of the logit spread observed for examinee proficiency measures (14.93 logits). Thus, despite all efforts at achieving high rater agreement during extensive training sessions, the rater severity measures were far from being homogeneous. This striking lack of consensus among raters would have a considerable impact on decisions about examinee proficiency levels.

---

5 Examinees with extreme scores, that is, with minimum or maximum total scores, are not shown here (9 examinees had *below TDN 3* on all criteria, exactly the same number of examinees had *TDN 5* on all criteria); one of these examinees received extreme scores through the third ratings as well. As a result, non-extreme scores were available for 1,833 responses.

Fig. 4.1: Wright map from the many-facet rating scale analysis. Each star in the second column represents three examinees, and a dot represents one or two examinees. LR = linguistic realization. TF = task fulfillment. GI = global impression. The horizontal dashed lines in the rightmost column indicate the category threshold measures.

Logit	Examinees	Raters	Criteria	TDN Scale
	High	*Severe*	*Difficult*	(TDN 5)
	.			
7				
	.			
6	*.			
	*.			
	*.			
5	*			
	.			
	**			
4	***.			
	**.			-----
	**.			
3	**.			
	***			
	***	16		
2	*******.	13		
	***.	14		TDN 4
	***.	09 15		
1	*****	05		
	***.		LR	
	****.	04	TF	
0	***	06 08 11		-----
	*******	18		
	***.	17		
-1	***.	10 12	GI	
	***	02		
	****			
-2	**.	03		TDN 3
	**.	01 07		
	**.			
-3	**.			
	*.			
	**.			-----
-4	.			
	.			
	.			
-5	*			
	.			
	.			
-6	.			
	.			
	Low	*Lenient*	*Easy*	(below 3)

The fourth column ("Criteria") compares the three scoring criteria in terms of their relative difficulties. Criteria appearing higher in the column were more difficult than those appearing lower. That is, the higher the difficulty measure of a particular criterion, the more difficult it was for examinees to receive a high score on that criterion. Clearly, then, *linguistic realization* and *task fulfillment* were similarly high in difficulty, whereas *global impression* was much less difficult.

The last column ("TDN Scale") maps the four-category rating scale to the logit scale. The lowest scale category (*below TDN 3*) and the highest scale category (*TDN 5*) both of which would indicate extreme ratings, are shown in parentheses only. This is because the boundaries of the two extreme categories are $-\infty$ (for the lowest one) and $+\infty$ (for the highest one).

The horizontal dashed lines in the last column are positioned at the *category thresholds*, or, more precisely, at the *Rasch-half-point thresholds*. These thresholds correspond to expected scores on the scale with half-score points (Linacre, 2006a, 2010b). Specifically, Rasch-half-point thresholds define the intervals on the latent variable in which the half-rounded expected score is the category value; that is, in the present case, the TDN level. For example, for an examinee located at the lowest threshold (i.e., at –3.66 logits), the expected score on the scale is 2.5. At the next higher threshold (i.e., at –0.06 logits), the expected score is 3.5. Between these two thresholds the half-rounded expected score is 3.0, the value referring to scale category 3, which is *TDN 3*.

4.3 Defining separation statistics

The distribution of examinee proficiency measures depicted in the variable map pointed to pronounced between-examinee differences in writing proficiency. This was not quite unexpected given the typical composition of the TestDaF candidature, ranging from beginners just trying their luck at the TestDaF to highly advanced learners of German coming close to native-language proficiency levels. As mentioned above, the logit spread observed for the rater facet would be much more a matter of concern.

To summarize observations like these, several group-level statistical indicators are available. These so-called *separation statistics* are computed for each facet specified in the model (Myford & Wolfe, 2003; Schumacker & Smith, 2007; Wright & Masters, 1982).

In the following, four particularly useful separation statistics are discussed with a focus on definitions pertaining to the rater facet (analogous definitions can easily be derived for the examinee and criterion facets). Subsequently, the statistics are applied to the sample data in order to assess the variability of measures within each of the facets. Note that the statistics are computed based on the construction of measures from the very same set of rating data. Hence, the results obtained are expected to converge on much the same general conclusions. Differences between statistics mainly refer to the specific information they summarize and to the kind of substantive interpretation they suggest.

The first statistic, the *rater homogeneity index*, provides a test of the null hypothesis that rater severity measures in the population are all the same, after accounting for measurement error (Hedges & Olkin, 1985; Linacre, 2014b). This fixed (all same) statistic is:

$$Q_J = \sum_{j=1}^{J} w_j(\hat{\alpha}_j - \hat{\alpha}_+)^2, \tag{4.1}$$

where

$$\hat{\alpha}_+ = \sum_{j=1}^{J} w_j \, \hat{\alpha}_j \Big/ \sum_{j=1}^{J} w_j \tag{4.2}$$

and $w_j = 1/SE_j^2$. The statistical symbol SE_j refers to the standard error that is associated with the estimate of the severity parameter for rater j (see also Section 5.1); the severity estimate is denoted by the ^ (the "hat") above the Greek symbol for parameter α.

Q_J is approximately distributed as a chi-square statistic with $df = J - 1$ (*df* is short for *degrees of freedom*; e.g., Hays, 1994). In practice, a significant Q_J value for a given sample of raters indicates that the severity estimates of at least two of the J raters in the sample are statistically significantly different. Q_J is very sensitive to sample size; hence, this index may reach, or exceed, the critical level of significance, particularly in large samples, even though the actual rater severity differences are fairly small.

When the null hypothesis of equal severity measures is rejected, the difference in severity estimates of any two raters j and k ($j, k = 1, \ldots, J, j \neq k$) may be tested for statistical significance. As proposed by Fischer and Scheiblechner (1970) in the context of examining data–model fit, the following index, an instance of the so-called *Wald statistics*, can be used for that purpose:

$$t_{j,k} = \frac{\hat{\alpha}_j - \hat{\alpha}_k}{(SE_j^2 + SE_k^2)^{1/2}}, \tag{4.3}$$

where SE_j and SE_k are the standard errors associated with severity estimates $\hat{\alpha}_j$ and $\hat{\alpha}_k$, respectively (see also Wright & Masters, 1982; Wright & Stone, 1979). The Wald statistic shown in Equation 4.3 follows approximately a *t* distribution with $df = n_j + n_k - 2$, where n_j and n_k are the number of ratings provided by raters *j* and *k*, respectively.

Another group-level separation statistic is the *rater separation ratio*. This statistic gives the spread of the rater severity measures relative to the precision of those measures; that is, the closer its value is to zero, the more similar the raters are to each other in terms of their severity.

To see how the rater separation ratio is defined, first let the "true" variance of rater severity measures be expressed as

$$SD^2_{t(J)} = SD^2_{o(J)} - MSE_J, \tag{4.4}$$

where $SD^2_{o(J)}$ is the observed variance of rater severity measures and MSE_J is the "mean-square measurement error", that is, the average of the rater measurement error variances:

$$MSE_J = \sum_{j=1}^{J} SE_j^2 \bigg/ J. \tag{4.5}$$

Thus, the "true" variance of severity measures is the observed variance of these measures adjusted (corrected) for measurement error. Forming the ratio of the adjusted variance to the average error variance leads to

$$G_J^2 = SD^2_{t(J)} / MSE_J. \tag{4.6}$$

Taking the square root of the ratio in Equation 4.6 yields the desired index, that is, the rater separation ratio:

$$G_J = SD_{t(J)} / RMSE_J, \tag{4.7}$$

where $RMSE_J$ denotes the "root mean-square measurement error" associated with rater severity measures. The G_J statistic indicates the spread of rater severity measures in measurement error units; it has a range from 0 to infinity. The higher the value of this statistic, the more spread out the raters are on the severity scale.

Using the rater separation ratio, one can calculate the *rater separation index*, which is the number of statistically distinct levels of rater severity in a given sample of raters, separated by at least three measurement error units. The rater separation index, also called the *number of strata index* (Wright & Masters, 1982, 2002), is given by:

$$H_J = (4SD_{t(J)} + RMSE_J)/(3RMSE_J) = (4G_J + 1)/3. \quad (4.8)$$

For example, a rater separation index of 3.1 would suggest that raters can be separated into about three statistically distinct levels or classes of severity. By the same logic, when all raters were exercising a similar level of severity, a separation index close to 1.0 would be expected; that is, all raters would form a single, homogeneous class.

The last separation statistic to be considered here is the ***reliability of rater separation index.*** This index provides information about how well the elements within the rater facet are separated in order to define reliably the facet. It can be computed as the ratio of the "true" variance of rater severity measures to the observed variance of these measures:

$$R_J = SD^2_{t(J)} \,/\, SD^2_{o(J)} = G_J^2 / (1 + G_J^2). \quad (4.9)$$

Rater separation reliability R_J represents the proportion of the observed variance of rater severity measures that is *not* due to measurement error.

The observed variance equals the "true" variance if and only if the error variance is 0. As a result, R_J is restricted in the range of 0 to 1. Thus, unlike the separation ratio G_J and the separation (number of strata) index H_J, the separation reliability suffers from a ceiling effect (see Schumacker & Smith, 2007; Wright, 1996).

Note that FACETS output provides both population and sample versions of separation statistics. Population statistics should be used when it can be assumed that the element list comprises the entire population of elements; otherwise, sample statistics should be used. In the following, population statistics are reported for each facet (the particular assessment administration was unique in terms of examinees, raters, and criteria involved).

4.4 Applying separation statistics

The analysis of the present three-facet sample data yielded the separation statistics shown in the lower half of Table 4.2. In addition, the upper half of the table gives the means and standard deviations of the examinee, rater, and criterion measures, as well as the mean standard errors of the respective measures, the root mean-square measurement errors, and the adjusted (true) standard deviations. As mentioned previously, the rater and criterion facets were centered, that is, these facets were each constrained to have a mean element measure of 0 (for non-extreme measures). Thus, the examinee facet was the only one that was non-centered in this analysis.

Looking first at the homogeneity index *Q*, it is readily seen that the results were statistically significant for each of the three facets: At least two elements within each facet had measures that differed in a statistically significant way. For example, at least two raters did not share the same value of the severity parameter, after allowing for measurement error.

Regarding the separation ratio *G*, the value of 3.16 for the examinee facet indicated that the variability of the examinee proficiency measures was about three times larger than the precision of those measures. The *G* value obtained for the rater facet showed that the variability of the severity measures was more than six times larger than their precision. Compared to the examinee and rater facets, the estimation of measures for elements of the criterion facet rested on a much larger number of observations (each difficulty measure was estimated based on 648 observations). Not surprisingly, therefore, these measures were estimated with a particularly low error component (i.e., *RMSE* = 0.08). Accordingly, the criterion separation ratio attained a value higher than the examinee or rater separation ratio.

Table 4.2: Summary Rasch Statistics.

Statistic	Examinees[a]	Raters	Criteria
M (measure)	0.51	0.00[b]	0.00[b]
SD (measure)	3.17	1.41	0.69
M (SE)	0.89	0.21	0.08
RMSE	0.83	0.22	0.08
Adj. (true) *SD*	2.63	1.39	0.68
Homogeneity index (*Q*)	3,070.5**	883.7**	207.0**
df	306	17	2
Separation ratio (*G*)	3.16	6.42	8.31
Separation (strata) index (*H*)	4.55	8.89	11.42
Separation reliability (*R*)	.91	.98	.99

Note. *RMSE* = root mean-square measurement error. [a]Examinees with non-extreme scores only. [b]The rater and criterion facets were each constrained to have a mean element measure of zero. ** $p < .01$.

The number of measurably different levels of examinee proficiency was provided by the examinee separation, or number of examinee strata, index. In the example, the value of this index was 4.55, suggesting that among the 307 examinees included in the analysis, there were about four-and-a-half statistically distinct classes of examinee proficiency. This nicely coincided with the four-category TestDaF scale; that is, the measurement system worked to produce at least as much reliably different levels of examinee proficiency as the TestDaF writing section was supposed to differentiate.

Particularly enlightening is the separation index computed for the rater facet. The value of 8.89 suggests that among the 18 raters included in the analysis, there were nearly nine statistically distinct classes of rater severity—far more than would be expected when adopting the standard view with its implied objective of employing raters drawn from a group that is as homogeneous as possible.

Concerning the criterion facet, the separation index attained a value greater than 11 and, thus, a value much greater than the number of criteria actually included in the analysis. This result indicates that the spread of the criterion difficulty measures was considerably greater than the precision of those measures. Generally speaking, high separation is caused by a large number of observations available for each element in the facet and/or a large "true" standard deviation of the measures for each element; in case of a large "true" standard deviation, extra elements could be added to close the "gaps" between widely dispersed element measures.

The last separation statistic listed in Table 4.2, the separation reliability *R*, has *differing* substantive interpretations depending on the facet considered. For examinees, this statistic provides information about how well one can differentiate among the examinees in terms of their levels of proficiency; that is, the examinee separation reliability indicates how different the examinee proficiency measures are. Usually, performance assessments aim to differentiate among examinees in terms of their proficiency as well as possible. Hence, *high* examinee separation reliability is the desired goal. For example, if one were interested in separating high performers from low performers, corresponding to an examinee separation ratio G_N equal to 2, an examinee separation reliability of at least .80 would be required; in this case, a maximum of three strata could be reliably distinguished along the proficiency scale (i.e., $H_N = 3$).

For raters, the interpretation of the *R* statistic is decidedly different. When raters within a group exercised a highly similar degree of severity, rater separation reliability will be close to 0. Viewed from the perspective of the standard approach to rater variability, *low* rater separation reliability would be the desired goal, because this would indicate that raters were approaching the ideal of being interchangeable. By contrast, when raters within a group exercised a highly dissimilar degree of severity, rater separation reliability will be close to 1. In other words, unlike interrater reliability, which (broadly speaking) is an index of how *similar* raters are with respect to their severity, rater separation reliability is an index of how *different* severity measures are. Thus, these two kinds of reliability indices must be clearly distinguished. In the present analysis, rater separation reliability was as high as .98, attesting to a marked heterogeneity of severity measures.[6]

By comparison, if one were to build on the standard approach to interrater reliability and computed a widely used group-level statistic, for example, Cronbach's alpha (e.g., Bramley, 2007; Haertel, 2006), which is formally equivalent to the consistency type of the intraclass correlation coefficient (see McGraw & Wong, 1996), the mean alpha value resulting for the present set of raters equaled .76. This value comes close to what in many practical applications would be considered acceptable (e.g., Nunnally, 1978; Stemler & Tsai, 2008), suggesting that raters were functioning almost interchangeably. But, as the rater separation and reliability statistics clearly demonstrated, this conclusion would be mistaken. Actually, traditional group-level reliability statistics often mask non-negligible differences within a group of raters, lulling those in charge of assessment programs into a false sense of security (for a similar discussion with respect to the level of rater pairs, see Section 5.4).

Finally, the criterion separation reliability provides information about how different the criteria are in terms of their levels of difficulty. When all criteria within a scoring rubric are intended to be similarly difficult, low values of this statistic would be desirable. Alternatively, when the set of criteria is intended to cover a wide range of performance features spread out across the underlying difficulty dimension, high values of this statistic would be desirable. Looking at Table 4.2 again, it can be seen that the criterion reliability separation was close to its theoretical maximum, which was mainly due to the relatively low difficulty measure estimated for *global impression*.

One final note on the concept of reliability as discussed here seems warranted. Specifically, the question may arise as to how Rasch reliability estimates obtained for the *examinee* facet relate to conventional estimates of test reliability provided

6 Regarding the rater facet, the separation statistics G, H, and R can easily be computed by hand based on the measurement results given in Table 4.2 (and using Equations 4.7 through 4.9). Small differences in the resulting values will be due to rounding errors.

within the framework of classical test theory (CTT; for detailed discussions of the CTT approach to reliability, see de Gruijter & van der Kamp, 2008; Haertel, 2006; see also Section 9.4). A view sometimes taken says that examinee separation reliability is analogous, or highly similar, to conventional (classical) test reliability indices such as Cronbach's alpha or Kuder-Richardson Formula 20 (KR-20).

However, the relation between both kinds of indices is far from being simple. Rasch and classical estimates of reliability will typically differ for at least two reasons. First, Rasch-based methods of reliability estimation utilize a linear, equal-interval scale (if the data fit the model). By contrast, classical methods usually compute reliability on the basis of non-linear raw scores; that is, these methods are merely based on the *assumption* of linearity—an assumption that only rarely can claim validity.

Second, Rasch-based methods of reliability estimation exclude extreme scores, that is, scores that are minimum possible or maximum possible scores attained by some examinee. For the present data, the minimum possible score is the observed average 2.0, representing *below TDN 3* on each criterion; the maximum possible score is the observed average 5.0, representing *TDN 5* on each criterion. Extreme scores are excluded from estimation since the standard errors associated with these scores are infinitely large, and since extreme scores contain relatively little information about an examinee's location on the latent dimension. By contrast, classical methods usually include extreme scores. Yet, extreme scores do not have any error variance. Therefore, their inclusion serves to increase the reported reliability coefficient (for a more detailed discussion, see Clauser & Linacre, 1999; Linacre, 1997c; Schumacker & Smith, 2007).

To the extent, then, that raw scores deviate from linearity and/or extreme scores prevail in a given data set, Rasch- and CTT-based reliability estimates will differ. These differences need to be taken into account when relating Rasch estimates of examinee separation reliability to Cronbach's alpha or similar CTT-based estimates of test reliability.

4.5 Global model fit

Rasch models are idealizations of empirical observations (Bond & Fox, 2015; Linacre, 1997b). Therefore, empirical data will never fit a given Rasch model perfectly. Generally speaking, with a sufficiently large sample (and a sufficiently powerful statistical test), empirical data will always appear to be flawed. In this sense, *any* model can be shown to be false (Fischer, 2007; Lord & Novick, 1968; Wu & Adams, 2013). Assessing the global fit of data to a model may thus easily turn into a futile endeavor. Hence, it is a reasonable strategy to explore a model's *practical utility* or *practical significance* (Sinharay & Haberman, 2014). That is, we need to know whether the data fit the model usefully, and, when misfit is found, how much misfit there is, where it comes from, and what to do about it.

In his discussion of the pragmatic function of (false) models in science, philosopher William Wimsatt (2007) pointed out:

> What models are acceptable, what data are relevant to them, and what counts as a "sufficiently close fit" between model and data is a function of the purposes for which the models and data are employed.... Any model implicitly or explicitly makes simplifications, ignores variables, and simplifies or ignores interactions among the variables in the models and among possibly relevant variables not included in the model. These omitted and simplified variables and interactions are sources of bias in cases where they are important. (p. 96)

It can be a fairly challenging task to identify the variables that are potentially relevant in a particular assessment context. Sound theorizing in the respective field of research can be of considerable help, but in the absence of theoretical guidance a researcher will have to start somewhere. Whatever the finally proposed model may look like, a model that does not include the relevant variables is likely to be of limited utility.

In keeping with the three basic methodological steps outlined in the introductory chapter, the least a researcher could do is to start with a tentative set of hypotheses concerning the variables, or facets, having an impact on assessment outcomes. Failing to do so and performing an analysis on the basis of an incorrectly specified model will produce unacceptable data–model fit in certain parts of the model. To improve the fit, it is a suitable option to closely inspect the deviations from model expectations, to identify possibly hidden facets, and to change the model specification accordingly. When the changes result in improved fit it is generally safe to conclude that a source of bias has been identified, and the overall usefulness of the model is likely to increase.

This suggests that indices of global data–model fit are much less informative than sometimes assumed (for detailed accounts of global fit statistics, see Embretson & Reise, 2000; Swaminathan, Hambleton, & Rogers, 2007). If a given set of observations *does* fit a model, it may simply mean that a researcher has not gathered enough data yet; if it does *not* fit the model, the analytic work begins, identifying the potential sources of misfit or bias, refining old hypotheses or forming new ones as appropriate, in order to finally come up with a practically (more) useful model. The process of stepwise evidence-based model development is just one example of how false models may improve our descriptions and explanations of the world (Wimsatt, 2007; see also Fisher, 1993).

Early versions of FACETS (first released in 1987) did not provide global fit statistics. Only later an estimate of global data–model fit was included (Linacre, 2014b; see also de Jong & Linacre, 1993). This estimate is based on a *log-likelihood chi-square*, computed as $-2 \times$ (sum of the natural logarithms of the model probabilities for all observations), with its approximate df = (number of responses used for estimation) – (number of parameters estimated). In the present analysis, the resulting chi-square value was 2,546.43 (df = 1,523, p < .001), indicating significant lack of global data–model fit. Yet, in light of what has been said before, this result comes as no surprise; it is rather what can be predicted for nearly any set of empirical observations.

An alternative approach to assessing global model fit is to examine the differences between responses that were observed and responses that were expected on the basis of the model. This approach may also greatly help to identify sources of possibly lacking data–model fit. Usually, the differences between observed and expected responses are expressed as *standardized residuals* (for a formal definition of standardized residuals, see Section 5.1.2). According to Linacre (2014b), satisfactory model fit is indicated when about 5% or less of (absolute) standardized residuals are ≥ 2, and about 1% or less of (absolute) standardized residuals are ≥ 3.

Considering the present sample, there was a total of 1,833 responses used for estimation of (non-extreme) parameter values. Of these, 100 responses (or 5.5%) were associated with (absolute) standardized residuals ≥ 2, and 4 responses (or 0.2%) were associated with (absolute) standardized residuals ≥ 3. Overall, then, these findings would indicate satisfactory model fit. Note, however, that such a result does not preclude that specific parts of the measurement system (e.g., particular elements of the criterion facet or categories of the rating scale) exhibit notable deviations from model expectations.

Table 4.3: Highly Unexpected Responses in the Sample Data.

Examinee	Rater	Criterion	Observed Score	Expected Score	Residual (Obs. – exp.)	Standard. Residual
048	01	GI	4	5.0	–1.0	–4.8
065	18	TF	2	3.9	–1.9	–3.9
277	14	TF	2	3.7	–1.7	–3.2
246	02	GI	4	4.9	–0.9	–3.1

Note. Highly unexpected responses are defined as responses associated with (absolute) standardized residuals ≥ 3. GI = global impression. TF = task fulfillment.

To illustrate the practical utility of the residual analysis approach to the issue of model fit, Table 4.3 lists the unexpected responses associated with (absolute) standardized residuals ≥ 3 as obtained for the present sample data.

For example, the first line shows that the rating for Examinee 048 assigned by Rater 01 on *global impression* was 4, representing *TDN 4*. Based on the model shown in Equation 2.11, the expected score was 5.0, yielding a difference between observed and expected score of –1.0, and a standardized residual of –4.8.

Unexpected responses usually provide a valuable source of information about the functioning of the elements involved. For example, when there is an accumulation of unexpected responses associated with a particular rater, this may indicate that the rater had specific problems with adhering closely to the scoring rubric. Alternatively, an accumulation of unexpected responses associated with a particular criterion may indicate problems in the way that raters understood and used that criterion.

Though there were only four observations that deviated strongly from model expectations, the data shown in Table 4.3 might suggest probing further into the differential usage of scoring criteria. Whereas high standardized residuals were obtained for *global impression* and *task fulfillment*, none of those were obtained for *linguistic realization*. As a reasonable next step in the evaluation process, one could specifically look at the four essays involved in order to find out more about the possible sources of that misfit. At a more general level, patterns of unexpected responses may set the stage for studying interactions between facets, a topic dealt with in some detail in Section 8.4.

5. A Closer Look at the Rater Facet: Telling Fact from Fiction

Instead of working on common ground raters often appear to vary considerably in terms of deeply ingrained, more or less idiosyncratic rating tendencies that threaten the validity of the assessment outcomes. This chapter addresses in detail the measurement implications of ineradicable rater variability, thus enabling researchers and assessment practitioners to separate facts about rater behavior from fallacious beliefs about raters functioning interchangeably. After pinpointing the precision of rater severity estimates, the focus shifts to the analysis of rater fit, including a detailed discussion of control limits for infit and outfit statistics. Further key issues of the present chapter refer to the study of central tendency and halo effects, and to the extent to which raters can be considered independent experts in the rating process. The chapter concludes with taking up again the topic of interrater agreement and reliability.

5.1 Rater measurement results

5.1.1 Estimates of rater severity

The preceding discussion has made it clear that the 18 raters under study differed greatly in their measures of severity. Let us now look at more detailed measurement results for each individual rater. Severity estimates, their precision, and other relevant statistics are presented in Table 5.1.

Table 5.1: Measurement Results for the Rater Facet.

Rater	Severity Measure	*SE*	MS_W	t_W	MS_U	t_U	Fair Average	Obs. Average	*N* of Ratings
16	2.40	0.30	0.93	−0.2	0.80	−0.6	3.00	3.03	60
13	2.09	0.20	0.82	−1.3	0.74	−1.4	3.08	3.11	123
14	1.83	0.18	1.10	0.8	1.09	0.6	3.15	3.45	129
15	1.21	0.22	1.39	2.3	1.43	2.4	3.32	3.58	84
09	1.21	0.17	0.81	−1.6	0.79	−1.5	3.32	3.39	141
05	1.05	0.19	1.12	0.9	1.06	0.4	3.37	3.37	123
04	0.29	0.23	0.89	−0.6	0.87	−0.7	3.60	3.72	72
11	0.16	0.26	0.75	−1.4	0.75	−1.4	3.63	3.54	57

Rater	Severity Measure	*SE*	MS_W	t_W	MS_U	t_U	Fair Average	Obs. Average	*N* of Ratings
08	0.14	0.18	1.05	0.4	1.07	0.5	3.64	3.49	141
06	0.09	0.20	1.11	0.8	1.08	0.4	3.65	3.59	102
18	–0.17	0.27	1.30	1.6	1.39	1.6	3.73	3.81	63
17	–0.57	0.18	0.81	–1.6	0.83	–1.1	3.83	3.98	135
12	–1.00	0.18	1.08	0.6	1.09	0.7	3.94	3.61	132
10	–1.02	0.19	1.02	0.2	0.99	0.0	3.94	3.48	123
02	–1.23	0.24	1.16	0.9	1.17	0.8	3.99	4.10	72
03	–2.01	0.19	0.82	–1.4	0.74	–1.0	4.17	4.02	123
01	–2.23	0.29	0.96	–0.1	1.23	0.8	4.23	4.52	60
07	–2.24	0.15	0.94	–0.5	0.92	–0.3	4.23	4.06	204

Note. MS_W = mean-square infit statistic. t_W = standardized infit statistic. MS_U = mean-square outfit statistic. t_U = standardized outfit statistic.

In the first column, raters appear in the order of their severity, that is, from most severe to most lenient. Each severity measure constitutes an *estimate* of a rater's "true" location on the latent variable. Thus, each measure is associated with some degree of estimation error.

The amount of error in a parameter estimate is given by its standard error (*SE*); the smaller an estimate's standard error, the higher its precision (de Ayala, 2009; Linacre, 2004a, 2005). As evident from Table 5.1, the *SE* values vary considerably between measures, indicating different degrees of measurement precision. Within the present context, *precision* refers to the extent to which the location of a given measure on the latent variable is *reproducible* based on the same measurement instrument or data collection procedure. Higher precision, or higher reproducibility, implies that we can be more certain about the value of the parameter in question (e.g., the "true" severity of a particular rater).

Standard errors can be used to define an interval around the estimate within which the value of the parameter is expected to fall a certain percentage of the time (de Ayala, 2009; Wright, 1995). Such an interval is called a *confidence interval* (CI).

For example, referring to Table 5.1, the severity measure of Rater 16 was estimated to be 2.40 logits, with *SE* = 0.30. Under the assumption of an approximate normal distribution, this rater's "true" measure is expected to fall within ±2*SE* around that estimate 95% of the time. For Rater 16, the CI has a lower limit of 1.80 (i.e., 2.40 – (2 × 0.30)), and an upper limit of 3.00 (i.e., 2.40 + (2 × 0.30)).

Note that the width of a CI represents the degree of uncertainty inherent in a set of data. Rater 16's CI has a width of 1.20, and thus is 0.40 wider than the CI for Rater 13, which is 2.09 ± 0.40, from 1.69 to 2.49. Hence, we can be more certain about Rater 13's measure than we can be about Rater 16's.

The CIs for Rater 16 and Rater 13 overlap strongly, which implies that their measures are not significantly different. As another approach to significance testing, the Wald statistic (see Equation 4.3) can be used. Not surprisingly, the severity difference of 0.31 logits fails to reach the level of significance, $t_{16,13}(181) = 0.86$, *ns*. By comparison, the difference between severity measures for Rater 14 and Rater 15, which is 0.62 logits, proves to be statistically significant, $t_{14,15}(211) = 2.18, p < .05$.

A large number of factors may contribute to a rater's tendency to rate more harshly or more leniently than other raters, including professional or rating experience, personality traits, attitudes, demographic characteristics, workload, and assessment purpose. For example, the most experienced or senior rater may also be the most severe because that rater may feel that he or she must "set the standard" for the other raters by noticing even small flaws in examinee performance that are otherwise likely to be overlooked. Conversely, less experienced or novice raters may tend to give the benefit of the doubt to examinees, especially when performance is at the border of two adjacent proficiency levels. In recent years, there has been a growing interest in studying the potential determinants of rater severity, mostly with the intent to inform rater training (e.g., Dewberry, Davies-Muir, & Newell, 2013; Eckes, 2008b; Leckie & Baird, 2011; McManus, Thompson, & Mollon, 2006; Myford, Marr, & Linacre, 1996; Stone, 2006; Winke, Gass, & Myford, 2013; see also Landy & Farr, 1980).

Reviewing the implications that well-documented differences in rater severity have for rating quality, McNamara (1996, p. 127) recommended "to accept variability in stable rater characteristics as a fact of life, which must be compensated for in some way". As explained earlier, rater training usually does not succeed in reducing between-rater severity differences to an acceptably low level. Therefore, in most situations, adopting the standard view that rater training needs to achieve maximal between-rater similarity, and eagerly pursuing this objective in rater training sessions, is extremely likely to end up in frustration of those in charge of the training.

The constructive alternative to striving after fictitious rater homogeneity is to accept rater heterogeneity within reasonable bounds and to adopt a suitable psychometric modeling approach. Many-facet Rasch measurement provides the tools to probe deeply into the complexities of rater behavior, and to use the insights gained for the purposes of making performance assessments as fair as possible. An important aspect of rater heterogeneity concerns the fit of each rater's ratings to the expectations that derive from the many-facet Rasch model employed in the analysis.

5.1.2 Rater fit statistics

The middle part of Table 5.1 presents statistical indicators of the degree to which raters used the TDN scale in a manner that is consistent with model expectations. These indicators are called *rater fit statistics*.

The study of rater fit is an indispensable step in investigating the accuracy of rater measurement results. As commonly understood, the accuracy concept makes reference to some external standard such as a set of expert ratings (Engelhard, 2013; Wind & Engelhard, 2013; Wolfe & McVay, 2012) or expectations derived from a specified model. In the present context, *accuracy* refers to the extent to which a given measure corresponds to Rasch-model expectations (Linacre, 2004a). Higher accuracy implies that we can be more certain about the *meaning* of the parameter in question. In other words, high measurement accuracy supports the validity of inferences and interpretations that build on the measures. Thus, highly accurate severity measures can be safely interpreted in terms of a given rater's tendency to rate consistently either too harsh or too lenient, relative to other raters or benchmark ratings.

Fit statistics compare model-based expectations with empirical data. More specifically, rater fit statistics indicate the degree to which ratings provided by a given rater match the expected ratings that are generated by the MFRM model. These statistics are formally derived below.

Let us first look at the exponential form of the three-facet RSM specified previously in Equation 2.11 (log odds version). According to the exponential form, the probability of examinee n receiving a rating of k ($k = 0, \ldots, m$) on criterion i from rater j is given by

$$p_{nijk} = \frac{\exp\left[k(\theta_n - \beta_i - \alpha_j) - \sum_{s=0}^{k} \tau_s\right]}{\sum_{r=0}^{m} \exp\left[r(\theta_n - \beta_i - \alpha_j) - \sum_{s=0}^{r} \tau_s\right]}, \tag{5.1}$$

where τ_0 is defined to be 0. The denominator in Equation 5.1 is a normalizing factor based on the sum of the numerators.

Let x_{nij} be the observed rating for examinee *n* provided by rater *j* on criterion *i*, and e_{nij} be the expected rating, based on Rasch parameter estimates. Differences between observed and expected ratings can then be expressed as *standardized residuals*:

$$z_{nij} = \frac{x_{nij} - e_{nij}}{w_{nij}^{1/2}}, \tag{5.2}$$

where

$$e_{nij} = \sum_{k=0}^{m} kp_{nijk} \tag{5.3}$$

and

$$w_{nij} = \sum_{k=0}^{m} (k - e_{nij})^2 p_{nijk}. \tag{5.4}$$

In Equation 5.4, w_{nij} designates the expected variation of the observed score x_{nij} around its expectation under Rasch-model conditions. This variation is called *model variance*. The model variance gives the amount of statistical information provided by an observation. Under the Rasch model discussed here, the amount of this information increases with increasing correspondence between the measures for examinee proficiency, rater severity, and criterion difficulty. The square root of the model variance, the denominator in Equation 5.2, is the *model standard deviation* (model *SD*, for short). Note that in the simplest case of the two-facet dichotomous Rasch model, the expected value becomes $e_{ni} = p_{ni}$, and the model variance becomes $w_{ni} = p_{ni}(1 - p_{ni})$.

Large standardized residuals for individual raters may indicate the occurrence of rater inconsistency. Standardized residuals with absolute values greater than 2 have $p < .05$ under Rasch-model conditions, and so indicate significant departure in the data from the Rasch model. Those observations are commonly considered significantly unexpected and may be subjected to closer inspection (Engelhard, 2002; Myford & Wolfe, 2003).

Squaring the standardized residuals and averaging over the elements of the relevant facets, residual-based indices of data–model fit are obtained. These summary statistics are called *mean-square (MS) fit statistics*. They have the form of chi-square statistics divided by their degrees of freedom (Smith, 2004b; Wright & Masters, 1982; Wright & Panchapakesan, 1969).[7]

To obtain a mean-square fit statistic for rater j, the squared standardized residuals are averaged over all examinees $n = 1, \ldots, N$ and criteria $i = 1, \ldots, I$, which were involved in the ratings by that rater:

$$MS_{U(j)} = \frac{\sum_{n=1}^{N} \sum_{i=1}^{I} z_{nij}^2}{N \cdot I}. \tag{5.5}$$

Equation 5.5 gives the *unweighted* mean-square fit statistic for rater j. The unweighted fit statistic is also called *outfit*. Rater outfit is sensitive to "outlying" unexpected ratings ("outfit" is short for "outlier-sensitive fit statistic"). Outlying ratings refer to a situation where the latent variable locations of rater j and the locations of the other elements involved, such as examinees and criteria, are farther apart from one another (e.g., separated by more than 1.0 logits). Thus, when a lenient rater awards harsh ratings to a highly proficient examinee on a criterion of medium difficulty, this rater's outfit will increase.

Weighting each squared standardized residual by model variance w_{nij} (as defined in Equation 5.4) leads to the following mean-square fit statistic:

$$MS_{W(j)} = \frac{\sum_{n=1}^{N} \sum_{i=1}^{I} w_{nij} z_{nij}^2}{\sum_{n=1}^{N} \sum_{i=1}^{I} w_{nij}}. \tag{5.6}$$

Equation 5.6 gives the *weighted* mean-square fit statistic for rater j. This statistic is also called *infit*. Rater infit is sensitive to "inlying" unexpected ratings. More specifically, infit is sensitive to unexpected ratings where the locations of rater j and the other elements involved are aligned with each other, that is, where the locations are closer together on the measurement scale (e.g., within a range of about 0.5 logits). Remember that variance w_{nij} indicates the amount of statistical information about the elements in question. Hence, infit is also said to be

7 Mean-square fit statistics belong to the class of parametric fit statistics, as opposed to non-parametric fit statistics that are not based on estimated Rasch or IRT model parameters (for reviews, see Karabatsos, 2003; Meijer & Sijtsma, 2001).

sensitive to unexpected ratings that provide more information ("infit" is short for "information weighted fit statistic"). Since such ratings are generally associated with higher estimation precision, infit is commonly considered more important than outfit in judging rater fit (e.g., Linacre, 2002c; Myford & Wolfe, 2003).

Infit and outfit mean-square statistics have an expected value of 1.0, and range from 0 to $+\infty$ (Linacre, 2002c; Myford & Wolfe, 2003). Raters with fit values greater than 1.0 show more variation than expected in their ratings; this is called *misfit* (or *underfit*). By contrast, raters with fit values less than 1.0 show less variation than expected, indicating that their ratings are too predictable or provide redundant information; this is called *overfit*.

Rater overfit often indicates the occurrence of central tendency or halo effects (e.g., Engelhard, 2002; Myford & Wolfe, 2004; for a detailed discussion, see Section 5.2). Moreover, in paired rating designs such as the one underlying the present data, overfit can also indicate when raters are colluding. For instance, if two insecure raters are paired together, they may consult, or imitate each other's rating style, in order to be "on the safe side". In a similar vein, when those in charge of rater training programs strictly follow the traditional approach, stressing the importance of high interrater agreement and possibly imposing a penalty for too much rater disagreement, raters may exhibit central tendency or try to agree with the ratings they think the majority of the other raters will provide. These rater tendencies will reduce the amount of information contained in the ratings and consequently lead to rater overfit.

Generally, misfit is more problematic than overfit, because misfit can greatly change the substantive meaning of the resulting measures and thus threaten the validity of the interpretations and uses that draw on these measures (Myford & Wolfe, 2003; Wright & Linacre, 1994). Moreover, it is advisable to study misfit *before* overfit, and to eliminate or reduce misfit, because this may help to make overfit disappear or become less pronounced.

Viewed from the perspective of behavioral strategies that raters may adopt, rater misfit can indicate an idiosyncratic rating style or otherwise overly inconsistent rating behavior. However, attention must also be paid to any occurrence of idiosyncratic examinee performance, which may actually be reflected in the ratings assigned.

Concerning the range of acceptable values for mean-square fit statistics, there are some guidelines that have been proposed in the literature. As a rule of thumb, Linacre (2002c, 2014b) suggested 0.50 as a lower-control limit and 1.50 as an upper-control limit for infit and outfit *MS* statistics. That is, Linacre considered mean-square values in the range between 0.50 and 1.50 as "productive for measurement" or as indicative of "useful fit" (see also Linacre, 2003b). Other researchers suggested using a narrower range defined by a lower-control limit of 0.70 (or 0.80) and an upper-control limit of 1.30 (or 1.20; e.g., Bond & Fox, 2015; McNamara, 1996; Wright & Linacre, 1994). It is commonly recommended to use *variable* critical ranges depending on the assessment context and the design or format of the assessment. For example, narrower ranges are deemed appropriate within high-stakes contexts like admissions testing or when studying objectively scored assessments like multiple-choice tests.

Defining an invariable, fixed range for values of mean-square fit statistics is not appropriate from a statistical point of view as well. The primary reason for this is that the variance of the fit statistics is inversely proportional to sample size (Wang & Chen, 2005; Wu & Adams, 2013); that is, the larger the sample size, the smaller the variance of the fit values.

In a simulation study, Wang and Chen (2005) generated data that conformed to the dichotomous Rasch model, varying the number of items and the number of persons. The results provided clear evidence of the sample size dependence of infit and outfit statistics. For example, when the data comprised 20 items and 100 persons, the values obtained for the infit statistic ranged from 0.66 to 1.41 ($M = 1.00$, $SD = 0.09$). By contrast, when the number of persons was increased to 800 (with the same set of items), the infit values only ranged from 0.86 to 1.12 ($M = 1.00$, $SD = 0.03$). As a consequence, quite a number of items in the smaller sample (100 persons) would be *incorrectly* identified as poorly fitting, given a lower-control limit of 0.70 and an upper-control limit of 1.30. The authors recommended adjusting critical ranges of fit statistics according to sample size.

A few years earlier, Smith, Schumacker, and Bush (1998) rather casually noted that Wright, through a personal communication (1996), had suggested (upper) critical values for the outfit mean-square statistic equal to $1+6\sqrt{N_r}$, and for the infit mean-square statistic equal to $1+2\sqrt{N_r}$. This suggestion has been taken up in the literature (e.g., de Ayala, 2009; Wolfe & McVay, 2012). In particular, Wolfe and McVay proposed to use the outfit upper control limit for the purposes of identifying rater effects.

More recently, Wu and Adams (2013) derived a simple expression for the asymptotic variance of the outfit statistic under the assumption that the data fit the (dichotomous) Rasch model. This variance is given by $2/N_r$, where N_r is the number of responses used for estimating the parameter of interest. For example, when estimating an item's difficulty, N_r is the number of examinee responses to that item; or, when estimating a rater's severity, N_r is the number of ratings provided by that rater.

To obtain a range of acceptable outfit values, Wu and Adams (2013) suggested using the formula

$$1 \pm 2\sqrt{\frac{2}{N_r}}. \tag{5.7}$$

In the present sample of raters, the number of ratings provided by each rater ranged from 57 (Rater 11) to 204 (Rater 07; see Table 5.1). Applying Formula 5.7 to these data, the critical range of outfit values for Rater 11 had a lower limit of 0.63 and an upper limit of 1.37; for Rater 07 the critical range was narrower, with a lower limit of 0.80 and an upper limit of 1.20.

Following Wu and Adams (2013), Table 5.2 presents asymptotic variances of the outfit statistic as well as lower and upper control limits for different sample sizes N_r. This table clearly demonstrates the sample size dependence of the critical ranges for outfit mean-squares. At the same time, the table illustrates that the statistic suggested by Wu and Adams can become much too demanding for very large sample sizes. As explained by J. M. Linacre (personal communication, January 29, 2015), a physical analogy is measuring our own heights with a micrometer (the unit of which is one millionth of a meter): the natural variation in our heights during the day would appear to be unacceptable. By the same token, use of Formula 5.7 may be reasonable only when running the first analysis of the data. After removing highly misfitting observations from the data set, the structure of the data changes and the outfit mean-square control limits computed according to the formula may become too strict; that is, the control limits may suggest misfit in the data that would be too small to have any meaningful impact on the measures (see also Linacre, 2010a).

More sophisticated statistical approaches to dealing with the sample dependence issue make use of bootstrap methods (e.g., Su, Sheu, & Wang, 2007; Wolfe, 2008, 2013). These methods estimate the unknown or analytically intractable sampling distribution of a statistic (e.g., fit statistic) through resampling with replacement from an empirical sample. Wolfe (2013) developed such a method to determine reasonable critical values for infit and outfit mean-squares. Su et al. applied bootstrap procedures to construct confidence intervals for evaluating fit statistics. Promising as these approaches may be, they have been developed within a limited two-facet assessment context. Research is needed that addresses bootstrap-based fit evaluation in a wider range of many-facet situations. Moreover, the issue of *meaningful* data–model fit discussed above is relevant here as well.

Table 5.2: Control Limits of the Outfit Mean-Square Statistic for Different Sample Sizes.

Sample Size	Variance	Lower Limit	Upper Limit
10	0.200	0.11	1.89
20	0.100	0.37	1.63
30	0.067	0.48	1.52
40	0.050	0.55	1.45
50	0.040	0.60	1.40
75	0.027	0.67	1.33
100	0.020	0.72	1.28
150	0.013	0.77	1.23
200	0.010	0.80	1.20
300	0.007	0.84	1.16
500	0.004	0.87	1.13

Note. Sample size is the number of responses used for estimating the relevant parameter. Variance is the asymptotic variance of the outfit statistic. Lower and upper control limits calculated according to Wu and Adams (2013).

Given the expected value and range of the mean-square fit statistics, it is clear that these statistics are non-symmetric about the mean. To provide a fit statistic that is symmetric about the mean 0 and whose values range from $-\infty$ to $+\infty$, the MS_U (or MS_W) statistic may be standardized using the Wilson- Hilferty cube-root transformation (e.g., Schulz, 2002; Smith, 1991). This transformation converts the mean square to a t statistic that has an approximate normal distribution. This t statistic is commonly referred to as a *standardized fit statistic*. In the present notation, t_U is the standardized outfit statistic, and t_W is the standardized infit statistic.

Standardized fit statistics can be used for the purposes of significance testing. Based on the standard normal distribution and choosing a conventional level of significance (i.e., $p < .05$), an absolute t_U or t_W value of at least 2 is commonly suggested to identify raters whose ratings warrant closer inspection. Significantly negative t values (i.e., $t \leq -2.0$) indicate rater overfit, significantly positive t values (i.e., $t \geq 2.0$) indicate rater misfit. According to Linacre (2003b), standardized fit statistics test the null hypothesis that the data fit the model "perfectly", whereas mean-square fit statistics indicate whether the data fit the model "usefully".

Referring back to Table 5.1, most raters had mean-square fit statistics that stayed within a narrowly defined fit range. Two raters (Rater 15 and Rater 18) showed a somewhat heightened degree of misfit, whereas Rater 11 exhibited a slight tendency towards overfit. In terms of standardized fit statistics, Rater 15 was the only one exhibiting a significant degree of misfit.

When testing fit statistics for significance, the issue of sample size dependence comes to the fore again: As sample size increases, ever smaller deviations from model expectations (i.e., $MS = 1.0$) will become statistically significant (Linacre, 2003b; Smith, Rush, Fallowfield, Velikova, & Sharpe, 2008; Wu & Adams, 2013). Hence, with sufficiently large sample size, the null hypothesis of perfect data–model fit will always be rejected. For example, items showing only a small misfit of $MS_W = 1.20$ would be flagged as significantly misfitting if sample size was well over 200 examinees; on the other hand, grossly misfitting items (i.e., items with $MS_W \geq 2.0$) would go undetected in samples of less than 10 examinees (Linacre, 2003b).

On a more general note, great care must be taken when using Rasch fit statistics to screen poorly fitting elements of a given facet, such as examinees, raters, tasks, or items. As simulation studies have demonstrated, the distributions of fit statistics are not only dependent on sample size, but also on various properties of the assessment instrument (e.g., test length, test difficulty), as well as on properties of the parameter distributions, such as the distribution of examinee proficiency or item difficulty measures (e.g., Karabatsos, 2000; López-Pina & Hidalgo-Montesinos, 2005; Smith, 1991; Smith, Schumacker, & Bush, 1998).

5.1.3 Observed and fair rater averages

Table 5.1 also displays statistics that help to gain a substantive interpretation of rater severity differences and their implications: fair average and observed average. Both kinds of averages are in the raw-score metric, that is, in the metric of the TDN scale.

An *observed average* for rater *j*, that is, $M_{X(j)}$, is the rater's mean rating across all examinees and criteria that he or she rated:

$$M_{X(j)} = \frac{\sum_{n=1}^{N} \sum_{i=1}^{I} x_{nij}}{N \cdot I}. \tag{5.8}$$

A non-trivial problem with observed averages is that they confound rater severity and examinee proficiency. For example, when a particular rater's observed average is markedly lower than other raters' observed averages, this could be so because the rater was more severe than the other raters or because the rater had more examinees of lower proficiency to rate. Fair averages resolve this problem: A fair average for rater *j* adjusts the observed average $M_{X(j)}$ for the difference in the level of proficiency in rater *j*'s sample of examinees from the examinee proficiency mean across all raters. Fair averages thus disentangle rater severity from examinee proficiency.

In order to compute a fair average for rater *j*, the parameter estimates of all elements of the other facets that participated in producing the observed scores, except for rater *j*'s severity parameter, are set to their mean values (Linacre, 2014b). In the present three-facet example, Equation 2.11 becomes

$$\ln\left[\frac{p_{jk}}{p_{jk-1}}\right]=\theta_M-\beta_M-\alpha_j-\tau_k, \tag{5.9}$$

where p_{jk} is the probability of rater *j* using category *k* across all examinees and criteria, and θ_M and β_M are the mean examinee proficiency and the mean criterion difficulty measures, respectively.

The *fair average* for rater *j*, that is, $M_{F(j)}$, is as follows:

$$M_{F(j)}=\sum_{r=0}^{m}rp_{jr}. \tag{5.10}$$

In the present sample data analysis, the rater severity measures, the range of which is theoretically infinite, are transformed back to the raw-score scale, which has a lower bound of 2 (rating category *below TDN 3*) and an upper bound of 5 (rating category *TDN 5*).

Fair rater averages enable fair comparisons between raters to be made in the raw-score metric. For example, comparing the fair averages of Rater 16 (the most severe rater) and Rater 07 (the most lenient rater), it would be safe to conclude that, on average, Rater 16 gave ratings that were 1.23 raw-score points lower than Rater 07 (see Table 5.1). That is, the severity difference between these two raters exceeded one TDN level.

5.2 Studying central tendency and halo effects

Until now the discussion of rater effects has almost exclusively dealt with the severity effect. One reason is that rater severity is commonly considered to be the most pervasive and detrimental rater effect in performance assessments. And since rater severity, as we have seen, can be parameterized in MFRM models, this effect is amenable to close scrutiny in the analysis of rating data. As mentioned earlier, however, other rater effects also need to be addressed in order to provide a more comprehensive account of rater variability (Barrett, 2005; Knoch et al., 2007; Myford & Wolfe, 2003, 2004; Wolfe, 2004, 2009). Foremost among these are central tendency and halo effects, both of which can be examined in a MFRM context by means of group-level and individual-level statistical indicators (Myford & Wolfe, 2004; Wolfe, 2009).

5.2.1 Central tendency

A rater is said to exhibit a *central tendency effect* (or *centrality effect*) when he or she overuses the middle category, or middle categories, of a rating scale while assigning fewer scores at both the high and low ends of the scale. Overuse of the middle categories leads to accurate ratings in the central range of the proficiency continuum, but results in ratings that overestimate the proficiency for low-performing examinees and underestimate the proficiency for high-performing examinees.

Central tendency is a special case of a rater effect called *restriction of range* (Myford & Wolfe, 2003; Saal et al., 1980). Restriction of range manifests itself by a narrowed dispersion of scores around a non-central location on the rating scale. For example, the ratings provided by Rater 01 discussed previously (see Table 3.4) clustered at the high end of the scale; that is, this rater only used the two highest categories of the four-category TDN scale. At the same time, the example illustrates that it may be difficult to distinguish between restriction of range and severity/leniency as separate effects (see Saal et al., 1980). Thus, in the example, Rater 01 may also be said to exhibit a strong leniency effect.

When a MFRM model of the kind specified in Equation 2.11 (i.e., a rating scale model) is put to use, information from scale category statistics may indicate whether the raters, as a group, showed a tendency to overuse the middle categories of the scale. For the present data, the frequency count and percentage of ratings that raters assigned in each scale category pointed to a general trend toward central tendency. Whereas the lowest category (i.e., *below TDN 3*) and the highest category (i.e., *TDN 5*) together were used in 30% of the ratings, the middle categories (i.e., *TDN 3* and *TDN 4*) were used in the remaining 70% of the ratings (see also Chapter 7, Table 7.2). Thus, there was a considerable imbalance in the spread of ratings across scale categories. As Myford and Wolfe (2004) noted, however, when only little is known about the actual distribution of proficiencies in the group of examinees under study, a clustering of ratings in the middle categories might as well reflect a real shortage of extremely low-performing and extremely high-performing examinees.

Further information on a possible group-level central tendency effect may be gleaned from the examinee separation statistics discussed earlier (see Table 4.2). When raters overused the middle categories of the scale, there should be a recognizable lack of variation between examinees in the proficiency measures estimated from the rating data. Thus, a non-significant homogeneity index, a low separation index, or a low separation reliability index, each computed for the examinee facet, would suggest a group-level central tendency effect (Myford & Wolfe, 2004). In the present analysis, none of the separation statistics indicated such an effect.

Criterion fit statistics provide another source of information that may be used at the group level. When raters overused the middle categories of the scale, there should be less variability than expected in the ratings on each criterion. Hence, criterion fit mean-square indices that are significantly overfitting would suggest the presence of a central tendency effect (Myford & Wolfe, 2004). Looking at the *MS* and *t* values shown in Chapter 7, Table 7.1, it can be seen that for each criterion the fit values stayed sufficiently close to the expected value (i.e., close to 1.0).

Central tendency effects may also be examined at the level of individual raters. In many situations, an individual-level analysis will yield more informative and more useful results than a group-level analysis, particularly when it comes to the implementation of rater training procedures. One potentially useful source of information is provided by rater fit statistics. If a particular rater exhibits centrality there should be less variation in his or her ratings than expected on the basis of the model. Therefore, rater overfit could be considered indicative of ratings clustered in the center of the scale; that is, mean-square fit indices should be much less than 1.0 (e.g., Smith, 1996). Though this is what is typically observed in the analysis of operational rating data, there may be conditions under which this will not be the case. For example, when scoring criteria differ widely in difficulty or when examinees differ widely in proficiency, mean-square fit indices greater than 1.0 can result even if a central tendency effect is known to be present (e.g., Myford & Wolfe, 2004; Wolfe, Chiu, & Myford, 2000).

In the light of this somewhat inconclusive evidence on the suitability of mean-square fit statistics for detecting central tendency effects, another statistical indicator that may be used at the level of individual raters is the *residual–expected rating correlation* ($r_{res,exp}$; Myford & Wolfe, 2009; Wolfe, 2004; Wolfe & McVay, 2012). Specifically, residuals are computed as the difference between the observed rating for examinee n by rater j on criterion i (i.e., x_{nij}) and the expected rating, based on MFRM model parameter estimates (i.e., e_{nij}; see the numerator in Equation 5.2).

When rater *j* exhibits a central tendency effect, the rater's ratings of high-proficient examinees are lower than the expected ratings; thus, the residuals are large and negative. At the same time, the rater's ratings of low-proficient examinees are higher than the expected ratings; thus, the residuals are large and positive. As a result, the residual–expected rating correlation for that rater (i.e., $r_{res,exp(j)}$) will be negative: High expected scores tend to go with large negative residuals and low expected scores tend to go with large positive residuals.

Based on the sample data, the residual–expected rating correlations computed for each of the 18 raters ranged from –.14 to .20; all of these correlations were weak and statistically non-significant. Hence, at the level of individual raters, there was hardly any evidence of a tendency to overuse the middle categories of the rating scale.

For the purposes of illustration, Table 5.3 and Table 5.4 display the rating scale category statistics obtained for two raters showing the lowest and the highest correlations in the sample, respectively: Rater 04 ($r_{res,exp(04)}$ = –.14) and Rater 11 ($r_{res,exp(11)}$ = .20). Note that the category statistics were computed based on a modified MFRM model discussed later (i.e., the rater-related three-facet partial credit model specified in Equation 8.2; see Section 8.3). As can be seen, Rater 04 used the two middle categories of the TDN scale (i.e., *TDN 3* and *TDN 4*) much more frequently than the other two categories; the middle categories accounted for no less than 82% of the ratings. Rater 11 made use of the middle categories in 68% of the cases—a value much more in line with the majority of the other raters.

The category statistics tables include two more sources of information relevant for detecting central tendency effects at the individual level: the mean-square outfit statistic and the category thresholds (see Myford & Wolfe, 2004). The mean-square outfit statistic compares the average examinee proficiency measure computed for each rating category and the expected examinee proficiency measure, that is, the examinee proficiency measure the model would predict for that category if the data were to fit the model. A central tendency effect would be signaled by an outfit statistic much greater than 1.0. As shown in the tables, the outfit statistics for both raters were reasonably close to the expected value of 1.0. Yet, the outfit values for Rater 04's middle categories were larger than the corresponding values for Rater 11, suggesting more of a central tendency effect in the ratings provided by Rater 04, as compared to Rater 11.

As mentioned before, a category threshold or, more precisely, a Rasch-Andrich threshold represents the point at which the probability is 50% of an examinee being rated in one of two adjacent categories, given that the examinee is in one of them. Now, if a rater exhibits a central tendency effect, he or she includes a relatively wide range of examinee proficiency levels in the middle category or categories. For example, the rater may consider the majority of examinees to cluster around an "average" proficiency level, when their actual proficiency levels are much more dispersed. In cases like this, the analysis will show that the category threshold estimates differ widely along the measurement scale.

Table 5.3: Category Statistics for Rater 04.

Category	Absolute Frequency	Relative Frequency	Average Measure	Outfit	Threshold	*SE*
b. TDN 3	3	4%	–3.15	0.8		
TDN 3	24	33%	–0.86	1.2	–4.16	0.66
TDN 4	35	49%	1.47	1.1	–0.07	0.35
TDN 5	10	14%	4.52	0.6	4.24	0.44

Note. Outfit is a mean-square fit index. Thresholds are Rasch-Andrich thresholds.

Table 5.4: Category Statistics for Rater 11.

Category	Absolute Frequency	Relative Frequency	Average Measure	Outfit	Threshold	*SE*
b. TDN 3	7	12%	–4.08	0.7		
TDN 3	23	40%	–1.71	0.6	–4.04	0.51
TDN 4	16	28%	2.26	0.7	0.58	0.47
TDN 5	11	19%	4.00	1.0	3.46	0.48

Note. Outfit is a mean-square fit index. Thresholds are Rasch-Andrich thresholds.

Compare again Rater 04 and Rater 11. The average distance between category thresholds for Rater 04 is 4.20 logits, for Rater 11 the average distance is 3.75 logits. Though being less than half a logit, this difference suggests that Rater 04 tended to include a wider range of examinee proficiency levels in the two middle categories of the rating scale. Taken together, Rater 04 showed some signs of a (weak) central tendency effect.

5.2.2 Halo

When examinee performance is rated using an analytic approach where assessments are made in relation to each of a number of criteria or features, halo effects may occur. Following common usage of the term, a *halo effect* refers to a rater's tendency to provide similar ratings of an examinee's performance on conceptually distinct criteria (e.g., Cooper, 1981; Saal et al., 1980). Halo effects may be due to at least three different cognitive or judgmental processes (see Fisicaro & Lance, 1990): (a) a rater's general impression of an examinee's performance has a similar influence on each criterion; (b) a rating on a particularly salient criterion has a similar influence on other, less salient criteria; (c) a rater fails to differentiate adequately between conceptually distinct features of the performance. Whatever the cause, or causes, in a given assessment context may be, the net result of halo effects is that examinees have less independent opportunities to demonstrate their proficiency.

The criteria used in analytic scoring are typically designed to represent distinct features, components, or dimensions of the construct that is of interest. Hence, it would not at all be surprising to learn from an analysis of the performance ratings that the criteria are correlated with one another. After all, the criteria, conceptually distinct as they may be, should work together in operationally defining the underlying construct. This poses a non-trivial problem for the detection of halo effects, since criterion correlations that are determined by the very nature of the criterion–construct linkage need to be distinguished from inflated correlations that are due to halo error. Murphy, Jako, and Anhalt (1993) used the terms *true halo* and *illusory halo*, respectively, to refer to the real overlap among the scoring criteria on the one hand, and the outcome of cognitive distortions, judgmental errors, and related construct-irrelevant factors on the other. The authors went on to note that it would be almost impossible to separate true from illusory halo in most applied settings. Using a rating design, however, that allows comparing scores obtained when raters evaluate examinees on *all* criteria to ratings obtained when each rater evaluates examinees on only a *single* criterion, may help to differentiate illusory and true halo (Bechger, Maris, & Hsiao, 2010; Lai, Wolfe, & Vickers, 2015). Now, with these caveats in mind, let us see how halo effects may be examined in a MFRM framework.

Group-level statistical indicators of possible halo error can be taken from the criterion measurement results. The rationale for this approach is as follows (Myford & Wolfe, 2004): When the majority of the raters were subject to halo error, the ratings would be highly similar across criteria and, as a result, the criteria would show only little variation in their measures of difficulty (presupposing that in fact there were substantial differences in criterion difficulty). Thus, a non-significant homogeneity index, a low separation index, or a low separation reliability index, each computed for the criterion facet, would suggest a group-level halo effect. For the present sample data, none of the separation statistics indicated such an effect (see Table 4.2). Yet, Myford and Wolfe (2004) rightly pointed out that an apparent lack of variation in criterion difficulty measures does not necessarily imply the presence of halo effects; that is, raters may be able to draw clear conceptual distinctions among the criteria (i.e., show no evidence of halo at all), yet, in the analysis, those criteria may prove to be similarly difficult.

At the individual level, statistical indicators that have been proposed as an aid in diagnosing halo bear on measures of rater fit (Barrett, 2005; Engelhard, 1994, 2002; Iramaneerat & Yudkowsky, 2007). However, use of fit statistics for that purpose is by no means simple or straightforward—not unlike the situation encountered previously when discussing ways to detect central tendency effects. Rather, as Myford and Wolfe (2004) made clear, halo can be signaled by rater infit and outfit mean-square indices that are significantly less than 1.0 *or* significantly greater than 1.0, depending on particular conditions of the measurement context. One such condition is the degree to which the criteria considered vary in difficulty. Low variation in criterion difficulty entails relatively small differences in expected ratings on those criteria based on the model. As a result, halo would be indicated by a pronounced rater overfit; that is, a given rater would provide ratings that appear highly redundant across criteria. Conversely, high variation in criterion difficulty entails relatively strong differences in expected ratings on those criteria based on the model. In this case, halo would be indicated by a pronounced rater misfit; that is, a given rater would provide ratings that appear highly unpredictable across criteria.

At the very least, thus, when examining the possible occurrence of halo effects, rater fit statistics must not be considered in isolation, separated from the broader measurement context. Moreover, it is advisable backing interpretations based on rater fit statistics by closely inspecting the pattern of ratings across criteria provided by grossly overfitting, or misfitting, raters, taking the degree of variation in criterion difficulty measures into account.

Another approach was suggested by Linacre (cited in Myford & Wolfe, 2004; see also Linacre, 2014b). According to this suggestion, the model used in the MFRM analysis would be explicitly matched to the specific kind of rater effect that is of interest. To the extent that a given rater fits that model, the rater may be considered exhibiting the rater effect in question. In the present case, all criteria would be anchored at the same difficulty, usually at difficulty 0. Following the rationale discussed above, raters whose fit values gravitate toward the expected value would be likely to demonstrate halo. Clearly, however, this approach presupposes that the criteria actually vary widely in difficulty; otherwise, anchoring them at the same difficulty would not make much of a difference.

Applying Linacre's anchoring method to the present sample data yielded negligibly small changes in rater infit and outfit. Remember that there were only three criteria, and two of them (i.e., *linguistic realization*, *task fulfillment*) were similarly difficult. The only rater who could possibly be suspected to exhibit halo based on a slight tendency toward overfit, as revealed in the original analysis (i.e., Rater 11, infit, outfit = 0.75; see Table 5.1), still had fairly low fit values of 0.77 (infit) and 0.80 (outfit) in the anchored analysis. The halo issue will be taken up again in Section 8.4.1. That section will present results from a Rater-by-Criterion interaction analysis, which is suited to shed more light on the nature of the rating tendencies exhibited by each individual rater.

5.3 Raters as independent experts

Viewed from the Rasch measurement perspective each score that a rater awards to an examinee is supposed to provide an independent piece of information about the location of the examinee on the latent dimension (e.g., examinee ability). More specifically, the estimation of model parameters in MFRM models is based on the assumption that the elements within facets are *locally independent*. Let us look more closely at this assumption.

As briefly discussed in Chapter 2, in a typical two-facet testing situation where examinees respond to a number of items that are scored either correct or incorrect, the assumption of local independence implies the following: For examinees at the same level of ability in the variable being measured, responses to any given item are independent of responses to other items on the test. Research has shown that an analysis that ignores possible dependence between items tends to overestimate the precision of examinee ability measures and may yield biased item difficulty parameters (Chen & Wang, 2007; Smith, 2005; Sireci, Thissen, & Wainer, 1991; Yen & Fitzpatrick, 2006). For example, tests of reading comprehension often contain items that are based on the same reading passage. These subsets of items, also known as *testlets* (Wainer & Kiely, 1987) or *item bundles* (Rosenbaum, 1988; Wilson & Adams, 1995), are likely to produce examinee responses that are locally dependent.

Carrying this logic over to the present three-facet situation, only by virtue of the fact that the *same* essay was rated by two (or more) raters, the ratings may be locally dependent to some extent. Technically speaking, in cases of multiple ratings of the same essays, raters are nested within essays in much the same way as items are nested within testlets (Patz, Junker, Johnson, & Mariano, 2002; Verhelst

& Verstralen, 2001; Wilson & Hoskens, 2001). Hence, local dependence becomes an issue to consider.

In general, when raters are asked to rate separately from each other, using their own expertise to assign scores to examinees, they usually show some level of disagreement. Part of this disagreement will be due to systematic factors (e.g., different levels of severity or leniency); part will be due to unsystematic or random factors, which can never be ruled out completely (e.g., fluctuations in physical testing or scoring conditions, changes in raters' attention due to fatigue, transcription errors, and many others). Nonetheless, raters, in particular trained raters who are subject matter experts, should be able to provide ratings based on much the same general point of view in terms of their understanding of the construct being measured (Linacre, 1997a, 1998a). This common ground, however, presumably adds to the local dependence of ratings.

Moreover, in some assessment contexts raters are required to stay close to a predefined level of agreement, and, when agreement falls below this critical level a number of times, the raters involved may be subjected to specific (re)training procedures or even be dismissed from the panel of operational raters (see Johnson et al., 2009). Penalizing raters for assigning discrepant scores typically entails a heightened normative pressure on raters toward unanimity; that is, raters will be motivated to achieve a high level of interrater agreement. Also, individual raters may gradually adopt a "play-it-safe" strategy, assigning more and more ratings in the middle categories of the rating scale; as a result, their ratings will show evidence of central tendency (see Wolfe, Myford, Engelhard, & Manalo, 2007).

The measurement implication of such a strict rater monitoring program is that the observations tend to violate the assumption of local independence among raters. Forcing raters into agreement and thus constraining rater independence by design is bound to enhance deterministic features in the ratings; that is, the amount of randomness in the data is substantially reduced. As a consequence hereof, instances of rater overfit occur more frequently, standard errors of parameter estimates are lowered, and the range of parameter estimates is markedly widened, which makes the judgments appear more reliable than they actually are.

In addition, trying to maximize interrater agreement can actually lead to reducing the validity of the assessment outcomes. For example, raters may settle for attending to superficial performance features that are easy to rate at the required level of agreement (see Hamp-Lyons, 2007; Reed & Cohen, 2001; Shohamy, 1995). Alternatively, raters may come to base their ratings, not necessarily consciously, on much the same criteria that are only partially explicit in the scoring rubric, as when rating grammatical accuracy of examinee performance on an assessment of communicative competence (McNamara, 1996). The net result in any case would be *construct under-representation*, which constitutes a major threat to construct validity (Downing & Haladyna, 2004; Messick, 1989, 1995). It may also be noted that this obviously unwanted effect is reminiscent of the attenuation paradox in classical test theory (Linacre, 1996b, 2002b; Loevinger, 1954).

In order to examine the extent to which raters in a particular scoring session acted as independent experts, or, alternatively, abandoned their independence and strived for a level of interrater agreement as high as possible, some statistical indicators produced by the computer program FACETS can be consulted (these statistics are requested using the "Inter-rater=2" command in the specification file; see Table 4.1). Since FACETS models raters as independent experts, raters are expected to show variation under identical rating conditions. Conversely, when raters act as "scoring machines" (Linacre, 1998a), they would be expected to provide identical scores under identical rating conditions.

One approach is to compare the *observed* proportion of exact agreements between raters under identical conditions (Obs%) to the *expected* proportion of exact agreements between raters under identical conditions (Exp%), where Exp% is computed on the basis of MFRM model parameter estimates. If Obs% is approximately equal to Exp%, then raters tend to behave like independent experts; if Obs% is much larger than Exp%, then raters tend to behave more like machines doing all of the scoring work (Linacre, 2014b).

To compute both kinds of proportions, the number of agreement opportunities needs to be known. For the present data, 273 essays were rated by two raters on each of three criteria, giving a theoretical maximum of 819 agreement opportunities (i.e., 3 agreement opportunities per essay); 34 essays were additionally rated by a third rater on the same set of criteria, giving a theoretical maximum of 306 agreement opportunities (i.e., 9 agreement opportunities per essay). There were 18 essays receiving extreme scores. These essays did not enter into the computation of actual agreement opportunities. Moreover, one of these essays was rated by three raters, giving a total of 60 agreement opportunities that were based on essays with extreme scores. Subtracting this number from the theoretical total of 1,125 opportunities gave 1,065 (actual) agreement opportunities.

The total number of observed exact agreements was 458; that is, Obs% = 43.0. The total number of expected exact agreements was 476.9, that is, Exp% = 44.8. Hence, Obs% was slightly smaller than Exp%. Overall, then, this indicated that the raters acted as independent experts.

At the individual level, most raters behaved pretty well in line with this general conclusion. The only exception to this pattern was Rater 15. The Exp% for this rater was 30.4%, whereas the Obs% was as high as 40.7%. That is, Rater 15, one of the more severe raters, showed much more exact agreements with paired Rater 07, the most lenient rater, than expected based on the model. It seems as if this rater tended to strive after agreement with what he or she thought to be something like the group norm, and in doing so at least partially deviated from his or her overall tendency to rate harshly. Quite in line with this reasoning, Rater 15 showed less model fit than any of the other raters in the group (see Table 5.1).

In addition, the issue of local rater dependence can be examined by means of a summary statistic that is conceptually similar to Cohen's (1960) kappa. Specifically, Linacre (2014b) suggested using the following Rasch version of the kappa index:

$$\text{Rasch-kappa} = (\text{Obs\%} - \text{Exp\%}) \;/\; (100 - \text{Exp\%}). \qquad (5.11)$$

Under Rasch-model conditions, this index would be close to 0. Rasch-kappa values much greater than 0 indicate overly high interrater agreement and, thus, a high degree of local rater dependence; large negative Rasch-kappa values indicate much less interrater agreement than expected based on the Rasch model, which may be due to unmodeled sources of variation in the ratings (e.g., hidden facets). Inserting the observed and expected proportions of exact agreements given above into Equation 5.11 yielded Rasch-kappa = –0.03. This finding corroborated the conclusion that, as a group, the raters in the scoring session considered here provided ratings that were sufficiently in accord with the independence assumption.

5.4 Interrater reliability again: Resolving the paradox

We are now in a position to relate the rater severity measures estimated in the present MFRM analysis to the rater consensus and consistency indices computed earlier (see Table 3.1). Particularly instructive are the severity measures for those raters belonging to one of the three rater pairs discussed in Section 3.2.3.

Figure 4.1 and Table 5.1, respectively, have shown that Raters 13 and 16 were located at the severe end of the logit scale. In fact, these raters were the two most severe raters in the group. The high reliability indices (consensus and consistency) observed for this rater pair (see Table 3.1 and Table 3.2) were thus due to their similar tendencies to rate examinee performance very harshly. Clearly, then, this is an instance of high reliability that must not be interpreted as evidence of accurate ratings; that is, on average, Raters 13 and 16 strongly *underestimated* the language proficiency of examinees in their respective samples, as compared to the other raters.

Considering the location of Rater 13 in relation to that of Rater 03, it is evident that things are quite different. In fact, Rater 03 turned out to be one of the more lenient raters in the group. Hence, it is not at all surprising that these two raters disagreed in the majority of cases (see Table 3.3). The low consensus values reported for these raters were obviously due to pronounced severity differences. At the same time, this particular case demonstrates that the consistency indices which yielded moderately high values (see Table 3.1) actually worked to conceal the striking difference in both raters' views of examinee performance.

Finally, the severity measures that were estimated for Raters 01 and 14 similarly point to a strong rater severity effect. Whereas Rater 14 was among the more severe raters in the group, Rater 01 was highly lenient. As a result, at least part of the low reliability indices (consensus and consistency) observed for this rater pair (see Table 3.4) could be accounted for by marked severity differences between these two raters.

The considerable degree of rater variability and the ensuing problems for the interpretation of interrater reliability indices are by no means specific to the sample data studied here, neither are they specific to the TestDaF writing section. Rather, as discussed earlier, rater variability is a general, notorious problem of rater-mediated assessments. For example, studying rater performance within the context of a local computer-based English speaking assessment, Yan (2014) reported an overall Spearman rank correlation between ratings assigned by first and second raters equal to .73. This consistency estimate suggested that raters achieved a satisfactory level of interrater reliability. However, the results of a MFRM analysis of the same data revealed a completely different picture: The rater homogeneity index was highly statistically significant, the rater separation index was 12.30, and the rater separation reliability was close to its maximum (.99), indicating that the raters differed strongly in their level of severity. The pronounced degree of rater variability was also reflected in an overall value of the exact agreement index of only 38% (for a discussion of other illustrative examples drawn from diverse fields of application, see Section 10.2).

Another perennial aspect of the rater variability problem is that between-rater severity differences at the group level are highly resistant to change; that is, rater training that aims at achieving homogeneity within a given group of raters regarding their degree of severity or leniency, is, as a rule, highly unlikely to meet with success (see Section 3.1). Yet, well-designed rater training can be effective in terms of increasing within-rater consistency and reducing extreme levels of rater severity or leniency (e.g., Carlsen, 2009; Elder et al., 2005; Weigle, 1998; Wigglesworth, 1993).

Given that within-rater consistency is sufficiently high, an efficient way to compensate for rater differences in severity is to compute, for each examinee, a fair score based on many-facet Rasch model parameter estimates. How this can be done is discussed in the next chapter.

6. Analyzing the Examinee Facet: From Ratings to Fair Scores

Observed scores in most instances should not be taken at face value. This is especially important when high-stakes decisions about examinees are involved. The present chapter deals with measurement results for the examinee facet, focusing on ways to ensure fairness of the assessment under conditions of substantial rater variability. Building again on the sample data, the chapter first illustrates the use and interpretation of examinee fit statistics and then goes on to elaborate on the adjustment of observed scores in order to compensate for between-rater severity differences. It is argued that adjusted or fair scores more dependably reflect examinee proficiency, and do so both at the aggregate score level and at the level of individual criterion ratings.

6.1 Examinee measurement results

As shown in the Wright map (Figure 4.1), there was a wide variation in examinees' writing proficiency. The estimates of proficiency measures had a 14.93-logit spread, which was more than three times larger than the logit spread observed for rater severity estimates (4.64 logits). Moreover, separation statistics confirmed that the examinees were well-differentiated according to their level of writing proficiency: The examinee separation or strata index was 4.55, with an examinee separation reliability of .91 (see Table 4.2).

In addition to the statistics presented earlier, FACETS provided a statistic testing the hypothesis that the examinee proficiency measures were a random sample from a normal distribution. This statistic took the form of a random (normal) chi-square statistic with $df = N - 2$. The result was a non-significant value of 283.8 ($df = 305, p = .80$), which supported the hypothesis of normally distributed proficiency measures.

Table 6.1 presents a portion of the measurement results for examinees selected from the present analysis. In the first column of this table, examinees appear in the order of their proficiency measures, that is, from more proficient to less proficient. The amount of estimation error associated with each measure, that is, its standard error (*SE*), is shown in the third column.

The number of observations, or responses, used for estimating proficiency measures was relatively small; for each examinee, there were only six ratings (by two raters) or nine ratings (by three raters). Therefore, the precision of estimates was considerably lower than that achieved for raters or criteria. For example, the average *SE* for proficiency estimates (0.89) was more than four times larger than the average *SE* for severity estimates (0.21; see Table 4.2). As a result, there is much less certainty about an examinee's "true" proficiency than about a rater's "true" severity. To illustrate, using the standard error of Examinee's 111 proficiency estimate (5.38 logits, *SE* = 0.81) to define a 95% CI, we find a lower limit of 3.76 (i.e., 5.38 – (2 × 0.81)), and an upper limit of 7.00 (i.e., 5.38 + (2 × 0.81)); that is, this examinee's "true" measure is expected to fall between 3.76 logits and 7.00 logits 95% of the time. The width of this interval is 3.24 logits, which is far more than the width of any of the intervals for rater severity measures.

Lower precision of estimates also implies that the difference between two estimates minimally required for reaching statistical significance increases. Adapting the Wald statistic (see Equation 4.3) to the purpose of comparing proficiency estimates of any two examinees n and m ($n, m = 1, \ldots, N, n \neq m$) gives:

$$t_{n,m} = \frac{\hat{\theta}_n - \hat{\theta}_m}{(SE_n^2 + SE_m^2)^{1/2}}, \qquad (6.1)$$

where SE_n and SE_m are the standard errors associated with proficiency estimates $\hat{\theta}_n$ and $\hat{\theta}_m$, respectively. The Wald statistic shown in Equation 6.1 follows approximately a t distribution with $df = u_n + u_m - 2$, where u_n and u_m are the number of ratings assigned to examinees n and m, respectively.

Table 6.1: Measurement Results for the Examinee Facet (Illustrative Examples).

Examinee	Proficiency Measure	*SE*	MS_W	t_W	MS_U	t_U	Fair Average	Obs. Average	*N* of Ratings
111	5.38	0.81	0.94	0.0	0.95	0.0	4.84	4.33	6
091	4.12	0.83	1.24	0.6	1.23	0.5	4.59	4.33	6
176	2.79	0.81	0.23	–1.8	0.23	–1.8	4.24	4.17	6
059	2.31	0.83	0.91	0.0	0.85	–0.1	4.12	4.50	6
213	1.29	0.79	0.70	–0.4	0.70	–0.4	3.88	3.83	6
234	0.18	0.81	1.88	1.3	1.87	1.3	3.58	4.00	6
179	–0.27	0.77	1.14	0.4	1.19	0.5	3.44	3.50	6
230	–0.46	0.80	0.39	–1.1	0.36	–1.2	3.39	3.83	6
301	–1.24	0.78	0.61	–0.7	0.59	–0.7	3.16	3.17	6

Examinee	Proficiency Measure	*SE*	MS_W	t_W	MS_U	t_U	Fair Average	Obs. Average	*N* of Ratings
052	−1.69	0.78	1.07	0.3	1.09	0.3	3.04	3.17	6
198	−1.78	0.78	1.16	0.4	1.16	0.4	3.02	3.17	6
149	−2.67	0.78	0.40	−1.2	0.39	−1.2	2.78	2.83	6

Note. MS_W = mean-square infit statistic. t_W = standardized infit statistic. MS_U = mean-square outfit statistic. t_U = standardized outfit statistic.

As an example, the proficiency estimates for Examinee 111 and Examinee 091 (see Table 6.1) differed by 1.26 logits; this difference was non-significant, $t_{111,91}(10) = 1.09$, *ns*. Moving down the measure column, the first significant difference between the estimate for Examinee 111 and any of the other estimates occurred for Examinee 059, $t_{111,59}(10) = 2.65, p < .05$; that is, these two examinees can be said to have different "true" writing proficiency.

Important as a detailed look at the precision of examinee proficiency measures may be, this is not the whole story. A careful evaluation of the measurement results for the examinee facet must also include a close inspection of examinee fit statistics, as this speaks to the issue of the accuracy of proficiency measures.

6.2 Examinee fit statistics

Examinee fit refers to the extent to which the ratings assigned to examinees are in line with expectations derived from the three-facet RSM specified in Equation 2.11 (or, alternatively, Equation 5.1). To compute a mean-square outfit statistic for examinee n, the squared standardized residuals are averaged over all raters $j = 1, \ldots, J$ and criteria $i = 1, \ldots, I$, which participated in producing the responses to that examinee's performance:

$$MS_{U(n)} = \frac{\sum_{j=1}^{J} \sum_{i=1}^{I} z_{nij}^2}{J \cdot I}. \tag{6.2}$$

Using weights that correspond to the model variance of the ratings (see Equation 5.4), the outfit statistic is transformed into the examinee mean-square infit statistic:

$$MS_{W(n)} = \frac{\sum_{j=1}^{J} \sum_{i=1}^{I} w_{nij} z_{nij}^2}{\sum_{j=1}^{J} \sum_{i=1}^{I} w_{nij}}. \tag{6.3}$$

As explained in the discussion of rater fit statistics, outfit is more sensitive to outlying unexpected ratings, whereas infit is more sensitive to inlying unexpected ratings. Therefore, other things being equal, examinee outfit will be greater than examinee infit when the unexpected ratings involve raters with severity measures located far away from the examinee proficiency measure. Conversely, when the raters are well-aligned with the examinee in terms of their locations on the latent variable, examinee infit will be greater than examinee outfit in case of unexpected ratings.

Table 6.1 presents the mean-square infit and outfit statistics, as well as the standardized fit statistics. According to the t_W and t_U statistics, none of the examinees included in the table showed significant misfit; that is, all (absolute) t values were smaller than 2.0. However, since sample size was small, a closer look at the mean-square fit statistics seems warranted. Most examinees were well in line with Rasch-model expectations (e.g., Examinee 052), whereas some examinees were overfitting (e.g., Examinee 176), and one examinee was misfitting (i.e., Examinee 234). Table 6.2 shows detailed fit analysis results for these three examinees.

The first column presents those two raters who provided ratings for each examinee; for ease of interpretation, the rater severity measures are given in parentheses, and the results for the more severe rater are shown above the results for the less severe rater.

Table 6.2: Detailed Results from the Fit Analysis for Three Examinees.

Rater (Severity)	Crit.	Obs. Score	Exp. Score	Residual (Obs. – exp.)	Model Variance	Standard. Residual	Combined Measure
Examinee 052							
08 (0.14)	GI	3	3.27	–0.27	0.29	–0.50	–0.86
	TF	2	2.89	–0.89	0.26	–1.74	–2.27
	LR	3	2.87	0.13	0.27	0.26	–2.37
12 (–1.00)	GI	4	3.61	0.39	0.29	0.73	0.28
	TF	3	3.19	–0.19	0.28	–0.37	–1.13
	LR	4	3.17	0.83	0.27	1.59	–1.22

Rater (Severity)	Crit.	Obs. Score	Exp. Score	Residual (Obs. – exp.)	Model Variance	Standard. Residual	Combined Measure
Examinee 176							
09 (1.21)	GI	4	4.18	–0.18	0.25	–0.35	2.55
	TF	4	3.84	0.16	0.25	0.31	1.15
	LR	4	3.82	0.18	0.25	0.36	1.05
17 (–0.57)	GI	5	4.64	0.36	0.24	0.73	4.32
	TF	4	4.27	–0.27	0.26	–0.53	2.92
	LR	4	4.25	–0.25	0.26	–0.48	2.82
Examinee 234							
10 (–1.02)	GI	4	4.09	–0.09	0.24	–0.18	2.17
	TF	5	3.75	1.25	0.27	2.42	0.77
	LR	4	3.72	0.28	0.27	0.54	0.67
07 (–2.24)	GI	4	4.40	–0.40	0.27	–0.76	3.39
	TF	4	4.04	–0.04	0.23	–0.09	1.99
	LR	3	4.02	–1.02	0.23	–2.12	1.89

Note. GI = global impression. TF = task fulfillment. LR = linguistic realization. Ratings on the TDN scale (i.e., observed scores) range from 2 (*below TDN 3*, lowest proficiency level) to 5 (*TDN 5*, highest proficiency level).

Compared to Table 4.3 presented earlier, information on two statistics has been added. The first statistic is the model variance (see Equation 5.4); dividing the residual by the square root of the model variance (i.e., the model *SD*) yields the standardized residual.

The second statistic is called *combined measure*. This statistic derives from an additive-linear combination of the measures of all the elements involved in producing a particular observation. In the present case, the relevant measure combination is specified by the three-facet RSM as defined in Equation 2.11.

Hence, the combined measure statistic $\hat{\omega}_{nij}$ for examinee n rated on criterion i by rater j is given by:

$$\hat{\omega}_{nij} = \hat{\theta}_n - \hat{\beta}_i - \hat{\alpha}_j \,. \tag{6.4}$$

For example, the proficiency estimate for Examinee 052 is –1.69 logits, the difficulty estimate for criterion *global impression* (coded as Criterion 1) is –0.97 logits (see Table 7.1, next chapter), and the severity estimate for Rater 08 is 0.14 logits.

Inserting these estimates into Equation 6.4 yields $\hat{\omega}_{52,1,8} = -1.69 - (-0.97) - 0.14 = -0.86$; this is the value of the combined measure that is modeled to produce the observed score (rating) "3" for this particular examinee. Note that the threshold parameter estimates are not included in Equation 6.4 because, within any given criterion, the set of threshold values is constant across observations.

The Pearson correlation between observed scores and combined measures provides additional information on the correspondence between observations and model expectations; in FACETS output this correlation is called *point–measure correlation* ("Correlation PtMea"; Table 7, Facet elements measurement report; Linacre, 2014b). When the scores awarded to a particular examinee are reasonably in line with the combined measures, the point–measure correlation is positive and high; in case of strong departures from model expectations, this correlation assumes negative values.

For a better understanding of the underlying relationships, the scores that each of the three examinees received were plotted against the combined measures, yielding the diagrams shown in Figure 6.1 (for a brief guideline on how to construct such diagrams, see Linacre, 2012). In each diagram, (shaded) diamonds represent scores provided by the more severe rater within a given rater pair, circles represent the scores provided by the less severe rater. To the right of each diagram, the results for examinee-related statistics are given: mean-square outfit (MS_U), proficiency estimate, and point–measure correlation (denoted by r_{pm}).

Let us first look at the measurement results for Examinee 052. The outfit statistic indicates close agreement between observations and model-based expectations (the same holds true for the infit statistic; see Table 6.1). Both raters provided ratings well in line with their estimated severity: Rater 08, the more severe rater, awarded an average score of 2.67, and Rater 12, the less severe rater, awarded an average score of 3.67; in fact, across the three criteria Rater 12's ratings were consistently one scale category (i.e., one TDN level) higher than Rater 08's ratings.

Fig. 6.1: Observed scores for three examinees plotted against combined measures modeled to produce them. The right-hand part shows examinee outfit statistics, proficiency estimates, point-measure correlations, and the two raters involved (the more severe rater listed first, the less severe rater second).

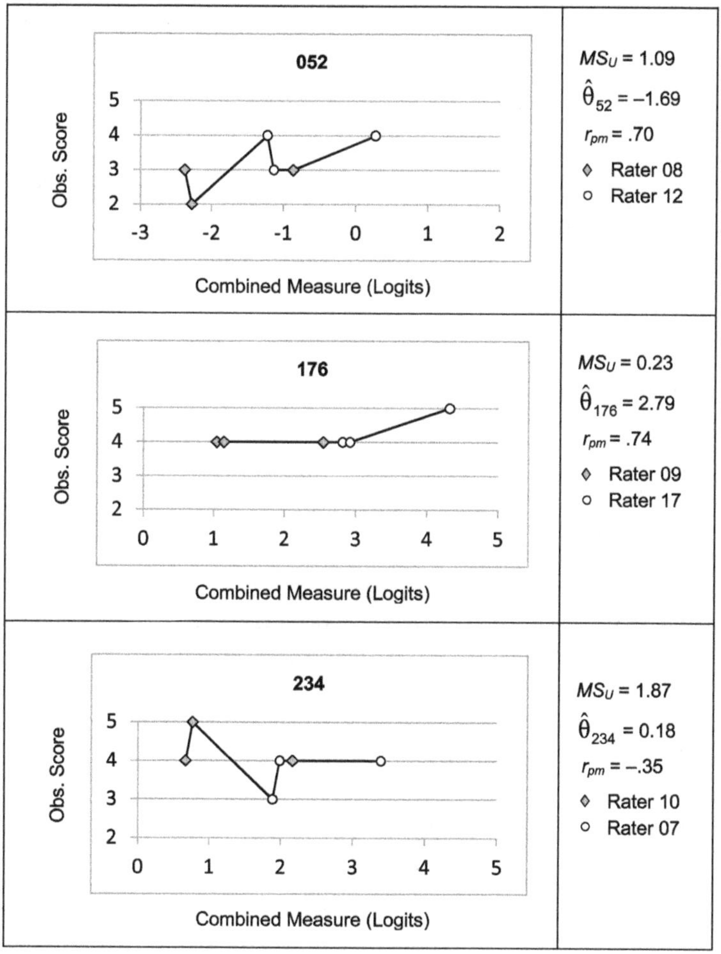

Though not constituting a significant departure from model expectations, relatively high standardized residuals were obtained for *task fulfillment* (Rater 08), where the observed score ("2") was lower than expected, and *linguistic realization* (Rater 12), where the observed score ("4") was higher than expected.

For Examinee 176, an overly smooth picture emerged: Both raters provided "muted" ratings, invariably awarding TDN 4, with one exception: Rater 17 awarded TDN 5 on *global impression* (the least difficult criterion; see Table 7.1, next chapter). Thus, there was much less variation in observed scores than expected, resulting in a small outfit statistic. Note, however, that overfit generally is more of a concern for psychometric analysis than for decisions in applied contexts: Overfit tends to stretch the measures along the latent dimension, to reduce their standard errors, and thus, to increase their reliability (or precision); yet, these measures will still be sufficiently accurate for most practical purposes.

The score–measure diagram for Examinee 234 shows a completely different situation: A relatively large outfit indicates that there was much more variation in the observed scores than expected. Hence, this examinee's proficiency measure appears to be inaccurate to a considerable degree. The cause for this inaccuracy is quickly spotted: Rater 10, the more severe rater, provided *at least as high* ratings for the examinee's performance as did Rater 07, the less severe rater; on *task fulfillment* and *linguistic realization*, Rater 10 even scored one TDN level higher. This striking departure from model expectations is reflected in a negative point-measure correlation.

What cannot be resolved by this kind of analysis is answering the question *why* Rater 10 provided such unexpected ratings for Examinee 234. But, of course, it is of great advantage to know which particular combination of elements (examinees, raters, and criteria) gave rise to significant data–model misfit. This knowledge is a prerequisite for taking steps to remedy the problem. Such steps may include discussing the departure with the rater or raters involved in an attempt to pinpoint possible biases, having an expert rater rescore the examinee's performance, or removing the most unexpected ratings from the data set before conducting the final estimation of model parameters.

6.3 Examinee score adjustment

Rater severity differences in the order observed here can have important consequences for examinees. Particularly, when examinee scores lie in critical decision-making regions of the score distribution, the final scores awarded to examinees may be affected by apparently small differences in rater severity.

Within the present context, an examinee's observed or raw score is computed as the average of ratings across the two (or three) raters involved. By contrast, an examinee's adjusted or fair score is computed on the basis of the parameter estimates resulting from the MFRM analysis. Thus, in a way analogous to the computation of fair averages for raters, where proficiency differences between the examinees rated by each rater are taken into account, examinee fair scores compensate for severity differences between the raters rating each examinee. In other words, for each examinee, there is an expected rating that would be obtained from a rater with an average level of severity. The reference group for computing this average severity level is the total group of raters included in the analysis.[8]

Formally expressed, an observed average for examinee n is that examinee's mean rating across all raters and criteria producing each rating:

$$M_{X(n)} = \frac{\sum_{i=1}^{I} \sum_{j=1}^{J} x_{nij}}{I \cdot J}. \tag{6.5}$$

To compute a fair average (fair score, expected score) for examinee n, the parameter estimates of all elements of the other facets that participated in producing the ratings, except for examinee n's proficiency parameter, are set to their mean values (Linacre, 2014b). In the present example, Equation 2.11 becomes

$$\ln\left[\frac{p_{nk}}{p_{nk-1}}\right] = \theta_n - \beta_M - \alpha_M - \tau_k, \tag{6.6}$$

where p_{nk} is the probability of examinee n receiving a rating in category k across all raters and criteria, and β_M and α_M are the mean criterion difficulty and the mean rater severity measures, respectively.

The fair average for examinee n is then given by:

$$M_{F(n)} = \sum_{r=0}^{m} r p_{nr}. \tag{6.7}$$

Analogous to Equation 5.10, use of Equation 6.7 transforms the examinee proficiency measures, the range of which is theoretically infinite, back to the raw-score scale, which, in the present application, has a lower bound of 2 (rating category *below TDN 3*) and an upper bound of 5 (rating category *TDN 5*).

---

8 If there is reason to believe that the reference group of raters as a whole has been unduly harsh or lenient, or if only a subgroup of raters with known level of severity or leniency has been available, benchmark ratings or group-anchoring procedures can be used to compensate for any group-level severity effects (see also Linacre, 2014b; Lunz & Suanthong, 2011).

Equation 6.7 defines the so-called *test characteristic function* (TCF). The graphical representation of this function is the *test characteristic curve* (TCC; e.g., de Ayala, 2009; Yen & Fitzpatrick, 2006). Just as the item characteristic curve (ICC) discussed in Chapter 2, the TCC is an S-shaped curve (i.e., an ogive). This highlights the fact that the functional relationship between the measures and the fair (expected) scores is non-linear.

Figure 6.2 displays the TCC obtained for the sample data. For ease of presentation, the horizontal axis shows the examinee proficiency scale using a bounded range of –8.0 to 10.0 logits; the vertical axis gives the expected score along the TDN scale (i.e., the fair score).

As the dashed lines indicate, a score of 2.5 on the TDN scale is expected for an examinee proficiency measure of –3.66 logits, a score of 3.5 is expected for a measure of –0.06 logits, and a score of 4.5 is expected for a measure of 3.76 logits. The intervals on the vertical axis of Figure 6.2, which are demarcated by the (horizontal) dashed lines, define the *score zones* between expected half-score points. Along the proficiency scale, the dashed lines are located at the category thresholds, that is, at the Rasch-half-point thresholds. Hence, the intervals on the horizontal axis of Figure 6.2, which are demarcated by the (vertical) dashed lines, define the *measure zones* in which the expected score half-rounds to the category value of the TDN scale. For example, the measure zone from –0.06 to 3.76 logits matches the score zone from 3.5 to 4.5 expected half-score points; scores within this zone half-round to the expected score of 4.0, corresponding to TDN scale category 4. Note that the locations of the Rasch-half-point thresholds are identical to the locations indicated by the dashed lines in the rightmost column of the Wright map shown in Figure 4.1.

Fair examinee scores help to illustrate the deleterious consequences that may ensue when raw scores are taken at face value. A case in point is Examinee 111 (see Table 6.1). This examinee proved to be highly proficient (5.38 logits, *SE* = 0.81), and the six ratings he or she received showed satisfactory model fit; the observed average was 4.33. Using the conventional rounding rule, the final level awarded would have been *TDN 4*.

Fig. 6.2: Test characteristic curve.

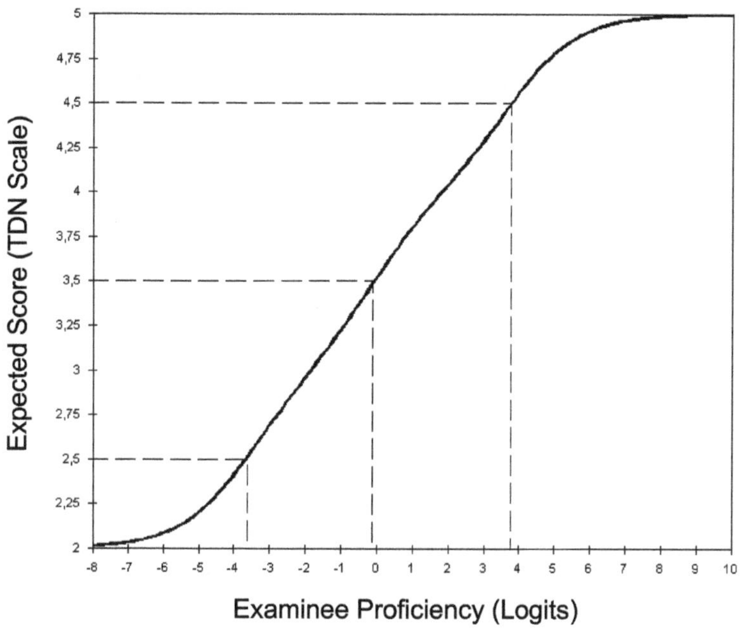

By contrast, this examinee's fair average computed on the basis of the estimated model parameters was 4.84, yielding final level *TDN 5* (i.e., the highest proficiency level on the TDN scale). Much the same *upward adjustment* of the final TDN level would have occurred with Examinee 091. Conversely, Examinee 059 and Examinee 230 would both have experienced a *downward adjustment*, if their fair averages were taken into account, as opposed to the observed averages.

This begs the question: Precisely what are the reasons for upward or downward adjustments of examinee proficiency levels? The data summarized in Table 6.3 help to provide the answer.

Table 6.3 shows which raters had been assigned to each of the examinees listed in Table 6.1. In addition, each rater's severity measure and the specific ratings he or she provided on each of the three criteria are presented. Also included are the TDN levels computed by means of model parameters (fair averages) or by means of the simple averaging rule (observed averages).

Table 6.3: Illustration of Examinee Score Adjustment.

Examinee	Rater	Severity Measure	Criterion Ratings GI, TF, LR (TDN*)	Fair Average (TDN)	Obs. Average (TDN)
111	13	2.09	4, 4, 4 (4)	**4.84 (5)**	**4.33 (4)**
	16	2.40	5, 5, 4 (5)		
091	14	1.83	4, 4, 3 (4)	**4.59 (5)**	**4.33 (4)**
	08	0.14	5, 5, 5 (5)		
176	09	1.21	4, 4, 4 (4)	4.24 (4)	4.17 (4)
	17	–0.57	5, 4, 4 (4)		
059	12	–1.00	5, 5, 4 (5)	**4.12 (4)**	**4.50 (5)**
	03	–2.01	5, 4, 4 (4)		
213	13	2.09	3, 3, 3 (3)	3.88 (4)	3.83 (4)
	03	–2.01	5, 5, 4 (5)		
234	07	–2.24	4, 4, 3 (4)	4.00 (4)	3.58 (4)
	10	–1.02	4, 5, 4 (4)		
179	17	–0.57	3, 4, 3 (3)	**3.44 (3)**	**3.50 (4)**
	11	0.16	4, 4, 3 (4)		
230	07	–2.24	4, 4, 4 (4)	**3.39 (3)**	**3.83 (4)**
	10	–1.02	4, 3, 4 (4)		
301	13	2.09	3, 3, 2 (3)	3.16 (3)	3.17 (3)
	03	–2.01	4, 4, 3 (4)		
052	08	0.14	3, 2, 3 (3)	3.04 (3)	3.17 (3)
	12	–1.00	4, 3, 4 (4)		
198	15	1.21	2, 2, 3 (2)	3.02 (3)	3.17 (3)
	07	–2.24	4, 4, 4 (4)		
149	17	–0.57	3, 3, 3 (3)	2.78 (3)	2.83 (3)
	11	0.16	3, 2, 3 (3)		

Note. TDN levels range from 2 (*below TDN 3*, lowest proficiency level) to 5 (*TDN 5*, highest proficiency level). Fair and observed averages that are associated with different TDNs for the same examinee appear in boldface. GI = global impression. TF = task fulfillment. LR = linguistic realization. TDN* = rater-provided TDN level. TDN = final TDN level.

Now it is plain to see that the upward adjustment of the TDN level for Examinee 111 came about because this examinee had happened to be rated by Raters 13 and 16, which, as we know from the analysis, were the two most severe raters in the group. Given that both raters provided consistent ratings (see the rater fit statistics shown in Table 5.1), it can be concluded that these two raters strongly underestimated the writing proficiency of that examinee, as compared to the other raters. This underestimation was compensated for by using the examinee's fair average.[9]

Likewise, the downward adjustment of the TDN level for Examinee 059 came about because this examinee had happened to be rated by Raters 12 and 03, which, as we again know from the analysis, were among the most lenient raters in the group. That is, these two raters overestimated the writing proficiency of that examinee, as compared to the other raters.

The level assignments for seven examinees remained unaffected by the score adjustment procedure. Yet, some of these cases are revealing about the problematic nature of rater severity similarities and differences. For example, Examinee's 213 fair and observed averages were highly similar (3.88 vs. 3.83), resulting in the same final TDN level (i.e., *TDN 4*). However, the raters involved (Raters 13 and 03) were located at opposing ends of the severity dimension, with TDNs as provided by these raters differing by no less than two TDN levels. Here, pronounced between-rater severity differences cancelled each other out, making the net result look pretty much like a fair TDN level. It is not hard to imagine what the result would have been if Examinee 213 had happened to be rated by similarly severe Raters 13 and 16 (which had been Examinee 111's bad luck).

The overall effect of adjusting examinee scores for variations in rater severity across all examinees can be illustrated by a scatter diagram that plots fair averages against observed averages (Lunz, Wright, & Linacre, 1990; McNamara, 1996). Figure 6.3 displays the *score adjustment diagram* obtained for the present sample of examinees.

Fair and observed averages were highly correlated (Pearson's $r = .96, p < .001$; Kendall's tau-b = .86, $p < .001$). Yet, in a notable number of cases, the differences between both kinds of averages were large enough as to have a critical impact on the assignment of final TDN levels. For example, given an observed average

---

9 With respect to the specific case of Examinee 111, Rater 16 provided less harsh ratings than Rater 13, although the severity estimate for Rater 16 was higher than that of Rater 13. Yet, both raters' overall severity estimates did not differ significantly. Moreover, Rater 16 tended to provide a greater number of harsh ratings at lower proficiency levels, particularly at level *TDN 3* (see Table 3.2, Section 3.2.3).

of 3.50, fair averages ranged from 3.04, suggesting *TDN 3*, to 4.09, suggesting *TDN 4*. Actually, in 53 cases (i.e., 17.3% of the sample) observed and fair averages would have led to differences in TDN assignments by exactly one TDN level (Cohen's weighted kappa = .81). The MFRM analysis therefore prevented a possible misclassification of about one-sixth of the examinee sample.

Fig. 6.3: Score adjustment diagram. Each dot represents an examinee with a given fair average (horizontal axis) and the associated value of the observed average (vertical axis). Dashed lines define critical score regions. Dots representing Examinees 111 and 230, respectively, are highlighted for illustrative purposes.

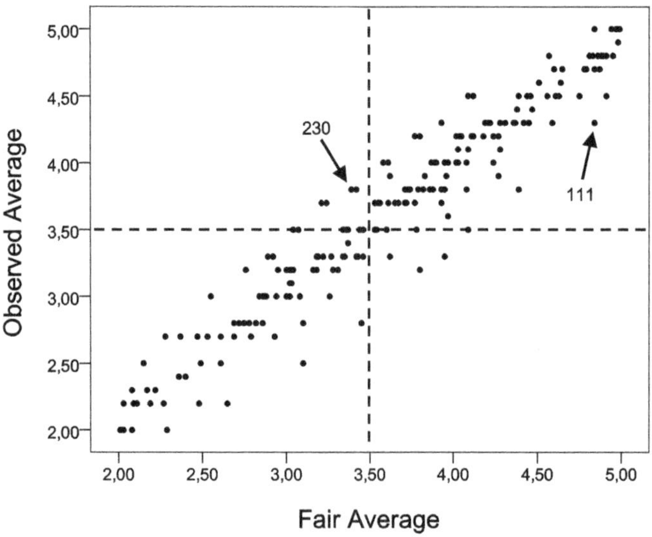

For the purposes of illustration, in Figure 6.3 dashed lines are drawn at fair and observed averages equal to 3.50. The intersection of the two lines at 3.50 creates four regions (or quadrants). The top-right and bottom-left regions show correctly classified examinees; these examinees would have been assigned to levels *TDN 3* or *TDN 4* by both fair and observed average.

By contrast, the top-left and bottom-right regions show incorrectly classified examinees. Thus, examinees located in the top-left region (e.g., Examinee 230) would have been assigned to *TDN 4* by observed average but to *TDN 3* by fair average. This corresponds to a downward adjustment in 22 cases (some examinees had identical combinations of fair and observed average and thus are represented by dots printed on top of each other). Conversely, examinees located in the bottom-right region would have been assigned to *TDN 3* by observed average but to *TDN 4* by fair average. This corresponds to an upward adjustment in 3 cases. Across TDN levels, there would have been 41 downward adjustments and 12 upward adjustments. As discussed at length earlier, the other examinee also highlighted in Figure 6.3 (Examinee 111) would benefit from an upward adjustment, resulting in the assignment of the highest proficiency level, that is, *TDN 5*.

Generally speaking, the horizontal spread of fair averages corresponding to each observed average shows the degree to which differences in rater severity obscure the meaning of an observed score, and the vertical spread of observed scores corresponding to each fair score shows the range of observed scores that an examinee of any given proficiency might receive depending on the rater or raters that happened to rate him or her.

The number of downward or upward adjustments ensuing from a given analysis, and the specific levels that will be affected by each kind of adjustment, usually depend on (a) the distribution of the observed scores in the sample of examinees under consideration, (b) the distribution of the severity measures within the group of raters, and (c) the number of categories contained in the rating scale and consistently used by the raters, that is, other things being equal, the higher the number of categories, the more adjustments are likely to result.

6.4 Criterion-specific score adjustment

The discussion so far dealt with score adjustments at the level of total scores (i.e., final TDNs). In many applied settings, however, it is desirable, or even mandatory, to compute and report adjusted scores at the level of individual scoring criteria or aspects of performance. Building on the sample data, this section illustrates how FACETS can be used to derive fair averages for each individual criterion entered in the analysis.

The basic procedure consists of four steps. In Step 1, a standard MFRM analysis is conducted to estimate model parameters, with an added command requesting to create an anchor output file. This output file contains specifications along with anchoring values for each and every parameter. In Step 2, the anchor file is modified in the criterion label section by commenting out all criteria but one, which is the criterion of interest. In Step 3, another MFRM analysis is run using the modified anchor file as a new specification file. This analysis produces measurement reports based on the selected criterion only, including the desired criterion-specific fair averages in the examinee measurement report. In Step 4, the adjustment procedure is restarted for the next criterion of interest, beginning with Step 2. The whole process ends when fair averages have been produced for the last criterion.

Table 6.4: Criterion-Specific Score Adjustment (Illustrative Examples).

Examinee	Fair Average (TDN)	Criterion-Specific Fair Average			*M* (TDN)
		GI (TDN)	TF (TDN)	LR (TDN)	
111	4.84 (5)	4.93 (5)	4.77 (5)	4.75 (5)	4.82 (5)
091	4.59 (5)	4.79 (5)	4.47 (4)	4.45 (4)	4.57 (5)
176	4.24 (4)	4.50 (5)	4.13 (4)	4.11 (4)	4.25 (4)
059	4.12 (4)	4.37 (4)	4.02 (4)	3.99 (4)	4.13 (4)
213	3.88 (4)	4.10 (4)	3.77 (4)	3.74 (4)	3.87 (4)
234	3.58 (4)	3.85 (4)	3.45 (3)	3.42 (3)	3.57 (4)
179	3.44 (3)	3.73 (4)	3.31 (3)	3.28 (3)	3.44 (3)
230	3.39 (3)	3.68 (4)	3.26 (3)	3.23 (3)	3.39 (3)
301	3.16 (3)	3.44 (3)	3.04 (3)	3.02 (3)	3.17 (3)
052	3.04 (3)	3.31 (3)	2.93 (3)	2.90 (3)	3.05 (3)
198	3.02 (3)	3.29 (3)	2.91 (3)	2.89 (3)	3.03 (3)
149	2.78 (3)	3.04 (3)	2.66 (3)	2.63 (3)	2.78 (3)

Note. TDN levels range from 2 (*below TDN 3*, lowest proficiency level) to 5 (*TDN 5*, highest proficiency level). GI = global impression. TF = task fulfillment. LR = linguistic realization. *M* = mean computed across criterion-specific fair averages. TDN = final TDN level.

In terms of the original FACETS specification file (see Table 4.1), the command to be added is "Anchorfile = W002_GI.anc". Placed, for example, right after the "Data file" command, this will create the anchor file "W002_GI.anc" for *global impression* (GI). Exclusion of the two other criteria is accomplished by commenting them out at the end of this file; that is, a semicolon is inserted before the criterion element numbers. Thus, "; 2 = TF, .4337068" is commenting out the criterion *task fulfillment*, and "; 3 = LR, .5324145" does so for *linguistic realization*. Then, running this anchor file, measurement reports will be constructed for *global impression* only. Note that the parameter value at which each criterion has been anchored in Step 1 (i.e., the estimate of the criterion difficulty parameter) is given after the criterion label as a number with seven decimal places.

Table 6.4 presents the results of this criterion-specific score adjustment procedure. For ease of comparison, each examinee's overall fair average and adjusted TDN level (taken from Table 6.3) are shown again in the second column. The next three columns each give the fair averages that are specific for each criterion and (in parentheses) the criterion-specific TDN levels. The last column shows the mean fair average computed across the criterion-specific fair averages (again along with the TDN levels); some of the mean values differ slightly from the overall fair averages due to rounding error (the TDNs are in perfect agreement, though).

Now it can be seen that Examinee 111 is highly proficient across all three criteria (*TDN 5*), whereas Examinee 091 is one TDN level less proficient on *task fulfillment* (*TDN 4*) and *linguistic realization* (*TDN 4*), respectively. The total adjusted score for Examinee 091 corresponds to the highest TDN level still, because the somewhat weaker proficiency on *task fulfillment* and *linguistic realization* is compensated for by this examinee's high proficiency on *global impression*. Much the same pattern is observed for Examinee 234, though at a level that is consistently one TDN lower.

More generally, criterion-specific score adjustments can be used to construct informative score or proficiency profiles. For example, in diagnostic assessment, where the aim is to identify strengths and weaknesses of examinees in a number of different performance features or skills, score profiles serve to provide criterion- or skill-specific feedback to examinees and thus may help to improve their weak points. A prerequisite for this usage of performance assessments is that the criteria or performance features were measured with sufficiently high precision and accuracy, and that the rating scale categories functioned as intended. These criterion- and scale-related issues are discussed more deeply in the next chapter.

7. Criteria and Scale Categories: Use and Functioning

Most often raters provide judgments using rating scales, where ordered categories are supposed to represent successively higher levels of performance. In analytic scoring, raters consider a given set of features of the performance of interest, and provide a separate score for each feature or criterion. In another approach, the holistic scoring, raters assign a single score to the whole performance. With each kind of scoring approach, raters need to distinguish between the different scale categories, awarding the score that best fits the performance at hand. In the case of analytic scoring they additionally need to distinguish between the different scoring criteria or subscales. The first section of this chapter deals with measurement results that are relevant to evaluating the functioning of a given set of scoring criteria. In the second section, differences between manifest and latent rating scale structures are pointed out. The final section presents statistical indicators of the usefulness and effectiveness of rating scale categories.

7.1 Criterion measurement results

In the sample data, *global impression*, *task fulfillment*, and *linguistic realization* were the elements of the criterion facet. Each criterion represented a distinct set of attributes that raters took into account when scoring an essay. One of the main goals of analyzing the criterion facet was to provide insight into the relative difficulty of the criteria, the precision of the difficulty estimates, and the degree to which the criteria worked together to define a single latent dimension.

Table 7.1: Measurement Results for the Criterion Facet.

Criterion	Difficulty Measure	*SE*	MS_W	t_W	MS_U	t_U	Fair Average	Obs. Average	*N* of Ratings
LR	0.53	0.08	0.97	−0.4	0.96	−0.5	3.52	3.53	648
TF	0.43	0.08	1.10	1.7	1.07	1.0	3.55	3.55	648
GI	−0.97	0.08	0.90	−1.7	0.91	−0.9	3.93	3.88	648

Note. LR = linguistic realization. TF = task fulfillment. GI = global impression. MS_W = mean-square infit statistic. t_W = standardized infit statistic. MS_U = mean-square outfit statistic. t_U = standardized outfit statistic.

A first view of the measurement results for the criterion facet was already provided by the Wright map. In Figure 4.1, the locations of *linguistic realization* and *task fulfillment* were close together and well separated from the location of *global impression*. Table 7.1 presents a more detailed look at the criterion measurement results.

Considering first the estimates of criterion difficulty, *linguistic realization* and *task fulfillment* were only 0.10 logits apart, indicating that it was similarly difficult to receive a high score on either criterion. By comparison, receiving a high score on *global impression* was much easier. Due to the large number of responses used for estimating difficulty measures (each estimate was based on 614 double ratings, plus 34 third ratings; last column in Table 7.1), the measurement precision was very high. In fact, the average standard error for difficulty estimates (0.08) was considerably lower than that for rater severity or examinee proficiency estimates (see Table 4.2). This implies that there was a high degree of certainty about a criterion's "true" difficulty. For example, using the standard error of the estimate for *linguistic realization* to define a 95% CI, we find a lower limit of 0.37 (i.e., 0.53 – (2 × 0.08)), and an upper limit of 0.69 (i.e., 0.53 + (2 × 0.08)), an interval only 0.32 logits wide.

An approximate t statistic analogous to Equation 4.3 (or Equation 6.1) confirmed that the difficulty measures for *linguistic realization* (coded as Criterion 3) and *task fulfillment* (Criterion 2) did not differ significantly from each other, $t_{3,2}\,(1294) = 0.88$, *ns*. By contrast, the difficulty measures for *task fulfillment* and *global impression* (Criterion 1) were highly significantly different, $t_{1,2}\,(1294) = 12.37, p < .001$.

As discussed before, issues of measurement accuracy are addressed by fit statistics. When considering criterion measures, an important question is whether the particular set of criteria used in the assessment is sufficiently homogeneous with respect to the latent dimension, that is, whether the criteria refer to the same dimension or whether they represent some other dimension (or dimensions) in addition to the intended, primary one. Such additional, or secondary, dimensions may reflect the influence of nuisance factors that are unrelated to the construct being measured or may actually constitute construct-relevant aspects of the performance. Whatever its source may be, the occurrence of multidimensionality threatens the validity of score interpretations and uses if not taken into account appropriately (for a detailed discussion of the dimensionality issue, see Section 8.2).

Criterion fit statistics are computed in much the same way as shown earlier for assessing rater or examinee fit. To compute a mean-square outfit statistic for criterion i, the squared standardized residuals are averaged over all examinees $n = 1, \ldots, N$ and raters $j = 1, \ldots, J$, which produced the observations on that criterion:

$$MS_{U(i)} = \frac{\sum_{n=1}^{N} \sum_{j=1}^{J} z_{nij}^2}{N \cdot J}. \qquad (7.1)$$

Criterion outfit is more sensitive to outlying unexpected ratings. The corresponding mean-square infit statistic that is more sensitive to inlying unexpected ratings is given by:

$$MS_{W(i)} = \frac{\sum_{n=1}^{N} \sum_{j=1}^{J} w_{nij} z_{nij}^2}{\sum_{n=1}^{N} \sum_{j=1}^{J} w_{nij}}. \qquad (7.2)$$

Table 7.1 presents the mean-square infit and outfit statistics, as well as the standardized fit statistics. For each of the three criteria, mean-square fit indices stayed well within very narrow quality control limits (i.e., 0.90 and 1.10). Also, according to the t_W and t_U statistics, none of the criteria showed significant misfit; that is, all (absolute) t values were smaller than 2.0. Hence, the criterion fit analysis confirmed the assumption of unidimensional measurement as implied by the Rasch model.

For the sake of completeness, Table 7.1 also lists fair and observed averages. Since all raters used all criteria to rate examinee performance, differences between both kinds of averages are due to rounding error.

7.2 Rating scale structure

In line with common practice, the categories of the four-category TDN rating scale (i.e., *below TDN 3, TDN 3, TDN 4,* and *TDN 5*) were printed equally spaced and equally sized on a scoring form. Raters used this form to score examinee performance by marking the appropriate category for each individual criterion. The intention was to guide and facilitate the scoring process; in particular, to convey to raters that the four scale categories were of equal importance and that each successive category reflected more of the underlying proficiency. Figure 7.1 depicts a simplified, schematic version of the manifest TDN rating scale.

Fig. 7.1: The basic four-category rating scale as presented to raters.

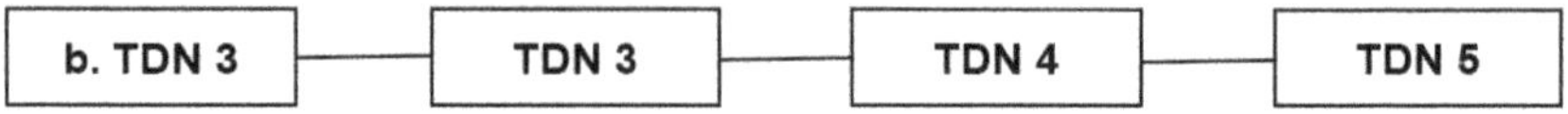

From a measurement perspective it is important to note, however, that it is an *empirical* question whether the locations of the categories define equal intervals along the latent continuum. That is, the ordering of rating scale categories must be considered a hypothesis about the structure of a given set of observations (Andrich, 2010; Andrich, de Jong, & Sheridan, 1997). The question then becomes: Did the raters in the operational scoring process interpret the rating scale as intended or did they perceive and use the scale in idiosyncratic ways, possibly manifesting significant deviations from scoring guidelines? Adopting a Rasch measurement approach, this question can be examined in due detail. Figure 7.2 depicts an example of the latent TDN rating scale structure as viewed from a Rasch perspective (a similar figure was presented by Linacre, 1999, 2004b).

Fig. 7.2: Hypothetical example of the four-category rating scale as modeled in a Rasch analysis (also shown are category thresholds τ_1, τ_2, and τ_3).

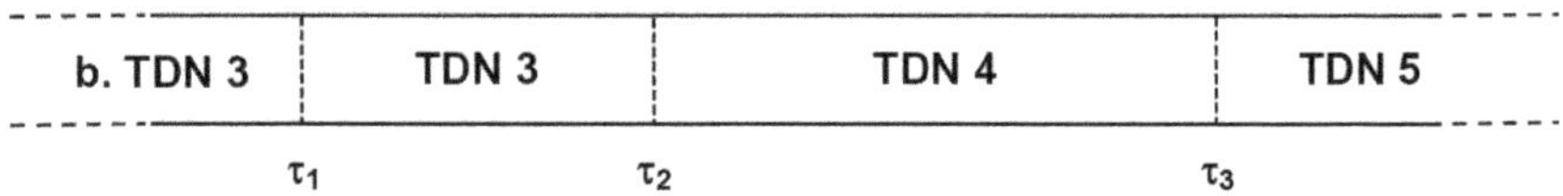

In Figure 7.2 there are two fundamental differences from the discrete category ordering shown in Figure 7.1. First, the two extreme categories are infinitely wide. This is because the latent variable is conceptually infinitely long, extending from $-\infty$ and $+\infty$. Accordingly, the bottom-level category *below TDN 3* (or whatever its label may be) does not have a well-defined lower boundary; and there will be examinees whose proficiency goes far beyond the top-level category *TDN 5*. Second, the size of the intermediate categories is variable, depending on how raters actually used the rating scale. In the example shown in Figure 7.2, the category representing *TDN 4* is wider than the one representing *TDN 3*. This illustrates the case that *TDN 4* covers a wider range of the latent variable; that is, *TDN 4* is used in a more inclusive way: performances assigned to this category show more variation than performances assigned to the more restrictive category *TDN 3*. In Figure 7.2, the boundaries between two adjacent categories are indicated by dashed vertical lines. The exact locations of these boundaries are given by the values of the Rasch-Andrich threshold parameter τ_k, which is estimated from the rating data.

7.3 Rating scale quality

As a preparatory step in evaluating the psychometric quality of rating scales, the orientation or polarity of each of the scales should be checked. Thus, before running a Rasch analysis of scale functioning, it is important to make sure that all scales are oriented in the same way as the latent variable under investigation; only then can higher ratings be assumed to imply more of the latent variable. When there are highly unexpected ratings or negative point-measure correlations associated with a particular scale, that scale should be closely inspected and possibly reversed or omitted from the final analysis. Not surprisingly, high positive point-measure correlations (.84 to .86) indicated that the present criterion scales were well-aligned with the latent variable (i.e., writing proficiency).

Based on Linacre's (1999, 2004b) suggestions, Table 7.2 provides an overview of indicators and guidelines for assessing the effectiveness of rating scale categories. In terms of Curtis and Boman's (2007) three-level x-ray analogy, these indicators provide a "micro-level" view at the data (where the "macro-level" refers to the test or assessment procedure as a whole and the "meso-level" refers to the items or criteria). Table 7.3 shows the rating scale statistics resulting from the MFRM analysis of the essay ratings.

Table 7.2: Rating Scale Quality Indicators and Guidelines.

Indicator	Higher Scale Quality	Lower Scale Quality	Remedial Action
Number (N) of responses per category	$N \geq 10$	$N < 10$	Omit categories, renumber categories sequentially
Response frequency across categories	Regular (uniform, unimodal, bimodal)	Irregular (highly skewed, unobserved categories)	Combine adjacent categories
Average measures by category	Monotonic increase with category	Reversals	Combine non-increasing, adjacent categories
Model fit of rating scale	$MS_U < 2.0$	$MS_U \geq 2.0$	Omit responses, combine categories, omit categories
Threshold order	Monotonic increase with category	Disordered thresholds	Combine adjacent categories
Size of threshold increase (logits)	≥ 1.4 and < 5.0	$< 1.4; \geq 5.0$	Redefine or combine categories; redefine or split categories

Note. MS_U = mean-square outfit statistic.

The first guideline refers to the number of observations or responses in each rating scale category. Linacre (1999, 2004b) recommended a minimum of 10 responses per category. Otherwise, category difficulties or thresholds may be poorly estimated and may prove to be unstable across similar data sets. In case of low-frequency (or unobserved) categories, remedial action consists of omitting these categories and sequentially renumbering the remaining categories.

Another guideline focuses on irregularities in the frequency with which the categories were observed. Table 7.3 presents the absolute observation frequency for each scale category in the second column. There is a peak in category *TDN 4*, with the next highest frequency observed in category *TDN 3*. Such unimodal distributions are generally unproblematic with regard to scale quality, as are uniform distributions where all categories are observed with similarly high frequency or even bimodal distributions peaking in extreme categories. By contrast, irregular distributions exhibiting a pronounced skewness or including a high number of intermittent low-frequency categories may signal aberrant use of scale categories. To remedy this problem, a reasonable strategy is to combine adjacent categories.

Table 7.3: Rating Scale Category Statistics.

Category	Absolute Frequency	Relative Frequency	Average Measure	Outfit	Threshold	*SE*
b. TDN 3	209	11 %	–4.13	1.0		
TDN 3	543	30 %	–1.19	0.9	–3.60	0.11
TDN 4	733	40 %	1.60	1.0	–0.10	0.07
TDN 5	348	19 %	4.29	1.0	3.70	0.08

Note. Outfit is a mean-square fit index. Thresholds are Rasch-Andrich thresholds.

A third indicator refers to the average measure by rating scale category, as shown in the fourth column (Table 7.3). This indicator is computed as the average of the combined measure statistics of all the elements involved in producing a rating in a particular scale category (for a formal definition of the combined measure statistic, see Equation 6.4).

The basic requirement is that average measures advance monotonically with categories; that is, higher average measures produce observations in higher categories, and *vice versa*. When this requirement is met, it is safe to conclude that higher ratings correspond to more of the variable being measured. As Table 7.3 shows, average measures increased strictly monotonically with rating scale category. When, however, average measures do not advance monotonically across categories or even demonstrate reversals, where lower average measures are associated with higher categories, serious doubt is cast on the usefulness of the rating scale. In cases like these, an option to consider is to combine non-increasing adjacent categories.

Rating scale effectiveness may also be examined through data–model fit statistics computed on a category basis. Thus, the category-related mean-square outfit statistic may be used to compare the average examinee proficiency measure and the expected examinee proficiency measure, that is, the proficiency measure the model would predict for a given rating category if the data were to fit the model perfectly. The greater the difference between the average and the expected measures, the larger the mean-square outfit statistic will be. In general, this statistic should not exceed 2.0. As Table 7.3 shows, the TDN rating scale had an excellent model fit; that is, values of the outfit mean-square statistic were equal, or very close, to the expected value of 1.0. In case of misfit, possible solutions include omitting highly unexpected individual observations, combining poorly-fitting adjacent categories, or omitting problematic categories altogether.

Referring back to Figure 7.2, a particularly instructive way to investigate the functioning of rating scale categories is to look at the ordering of the category thresholds. These thresholds, the Rasch-Andrich thresholds, should advance monotonically with categories: As one moves up the latent continuum, each scale category in turn should be the most probable (or modal) category.

Figure 7.3 provides a graphical illustration of the threshold order emerging from the sample data analysis. Specifically, the figure shows the *category probability curves* for the four-category scale that the raters used when rating examinees on the three criteria. The horizontal axis represents the examinee proficiency scale; the vertical axis gives the probability of being rated in each category. There is one curve for each category. The points along the horizontal axis at which the probability curves of two adjacent rating scale categories cross denote the Rasch-Andrich thresholds, as indicated by the dashed lines. For example, the probability curves of the scale categories *below TDN 3* and *TDN 3* cross at –3.60 logits, denoting the lowest of the three thresholds.

As shown in Figure 7.3, there is a separate peak for each category; that is, each category is in turn the most likely category along the latent variable. Put differently, each peak appears as a distinct "hill". Similarly, the category thresholds are nicely ordered from left to right: there is a clear progression of scale category thresholds from –3.60 logits (i.e., the threshold between categories *below TDN 3* and *TDN 3*) to 3.70 logits (i.e., the threshold between categories *TDN 4* and *TDN 5*). Table 7.3 presents the values of the threshold estimates and their associated standard errors.

By the way, Rasch-Andrich thresholds should not be confused with Rasch-half-point thresholds; the latter are defined on the latent variable in relation to expected scores instead of category probabilities (for comparison purposes, consider again Figure 6.2 showing the test characteristic curve and the associated Rasch-half-point thresholds). As a consequence of these different threshold notions, the values of Rasch-Andrich thresholds usually differ from the values of Rasch-half-point thresholds to some extent (see Linacre, 2006a, 2010b).

When the thresholds do not advance monotonically with categories, that is, when the thresholds are disordered, it can be inferred that the rating scale does not function properly: As one moves up the latent continuum, the categories involved would never be the most likely response to be observed (e.g., Tennant, 2004; but see also Linacre, 2010b). Note, however, that the requirement of ordered thresholds is not part of the mathematical structure of polytomous Rasch models such as the RSM or the PCM (e.g., Luo, 2005; Verhelst & Verstralen, 2008).

Fig. 7.3: Category probability curves for the TDN rating scale.

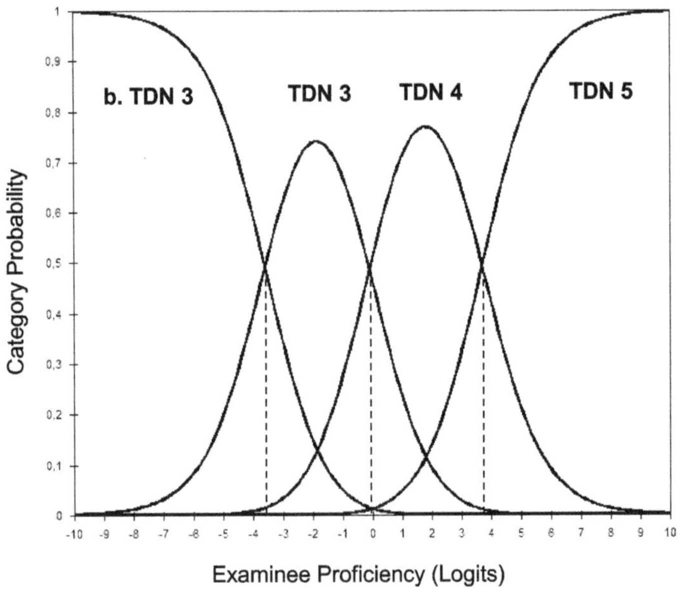

The last scale quality criterion shown in Table 7.2 refers to the size of the increase in category threshold values: The thresholds should advance by at least 1.4 logits; at the same time, they should advance by less than 5.0 logits (Linacre, 2004b).

As can be seen from the threshold column of Table 7.3, the distances between calibrations of adjacent categories all stayed within the range defined by these lower and upper limits.

When the thresholds are too close, the categories involved are presumably less distinctive than intended. For remedial action, one may consider to redefine, or combine, the categories to increase the range of performance covered. On the other hand, when the lower and upper boundaries of a given category are too far apart, the category represents a range of performance that is possibly much wider than intended, with only very few observations falling in the middle of the category. In this case, redefining the category as two narrower categories seems to be a viable option (Linacre, 2004b).

As suggested throughout the discussion of scale quality indicators, in case of problems with the functionality of a given rating scale, one remedy is to collapse adjacent categories and reanalyze the data. In principle, this can be done in a stepwise fashion until the optimal design of the rating scale has been found (for an example of such an iterative process of rating scale construction, see Smith, Wakely, de Kruif, & Swartz, 2003; see also Zhu, 2002; Zhu, Updyke, & Lewandowski, 1997). On a cautionary note, collapsing categories should not be based on statistical criteria alone, since each new category must be wholly interpretable in the light of the latent variable under investigation.

In addition, C. M. Myford (personal communication, February 24, 2015) warned against prematurely collapsing categories, in particular when the researchers are working with small samples of raters and/or examinee performances (or products) and have not yet had the opportunity to see the full potential use of that scale. In such studies it might be a better strategy to use the rating scales with larger samples of raters and/or examinees *before* deciding that a rating scale is not working in a satisfactory fashion.

8. Advanced Many-Facet Rasch Measurement

The many-facet Rasch model discussed so far has been concerned with basic issues of evaluating the quality of rater-mediated assessments. Each of the facets involved was analyzed in detail, including a first look at the structure of the rating scale. Yet, there is much more to a MFRM modeling approach than described in the preceding chapters. In particular, MFRM models can be tailored to fit a variety of assessment situations. In order to provide a brief overview of more advanced models, different types of scoring or scoring formats are presented first, followed by issues of measurement dimensionality. Then the focus is on the specific ways in which the rating scale was put to use, distinguishing between rating scale, partial credit, and hybrid models. Another section addresses the study of interactions between facets and introduces methods for the analysis of rater bias. The chapter concludes with a summary of MFRM models frequently encountered in the field of rater-mediated assessment.

8.1 Scoring formats

The data used to estimate the parameters of a particular facets model most often follow a polytomous format, as when raters score examinee performance based on a rating scale with three or four ordered categories. There are a number of other types of scoring that also yield data suitable for a MFRM analysis; first and foremost dichotomous scoring, as when examinees take a multiple-choice vocabulary test and their responses to each test item are scored either correct or incorrect, or when raters decide whether responses of examinees to short-answer questions in a note-taking task include or do not include the predefined key words.

Scoring formats much less common in language and educational testing contexts but nonetheless amenable to many-facet Rasch analyses comprise binomial trials or Poisson counts (Wright & Masters, 1982). *Binomial trials* are defined as situations where examinees are given a fixed number of independent attempts at an item or a task, and the number of successes or failures is counted (e.g., counts of reading or writing errors).

If the number of independent binomial trials is potentially infinite and the probability of success at each trial is small, then the resulting data may be modeled as *Poisson counts* (e.g., the number of words that an examinee can read correctly within five minutes). Finally, even a mix of different kinds of data, for example, dichotomous data, polytomous data, and binomial trials data combined in a single data set, can be used for the purposes of parameter estimation in a MFRM framework.

8.2 Dimensionality

As mentioned before, Rasch models are generally used to measure a single latent variable or dimension (e.g., examinee writing proficiency); that is, they are *unidimensional* models. This is not to say, however, that the construct being measured has to be unidimensional as well. Unidimensional measurement does not require that performance on a set of items, or ratings of examinee performance on a set of criteria, be due to a *single* psychological component, dimension, or process (see Bejar, 1983; Reckase, Ackerman, & Carlson, 1988). The requirement is only that the items on a test or the criteria on an assessment instrument work together to form a single underlying pattern of empirical observations.

It is thus important to distinguish between unidimensional measurement, also known as *psychometric* unidimensionality, and *psychological* unidimensionality (Henning, 1992; McNamara, 1996). In fact, ratings of examinee performance, especially ratings based on an analytic rating approach, usually incorporate a variety of performance features referring to a latent variable or construct, which for sound theoretical reasons may be considered a composite of abilities, rather than only a single ability. Moreover, as mentioned earlier in the discussion of global model fit (see Section 4.5), Rasch models are idealizations of empirical data. Hence, unidimensional measurement is also an idealization—but empirical data are never strictly unidimensional. Therefore, unidimensionality of a test or an assessment is not to be decided upon in a yes-or-no fashion; it is rather a matter of degree. In other words, the important question is whether departure from unidimensionality becomes so large that it threatens the interpretation of measurement results.

Within the context of Rasch measurement there are several approaches to testing for unidimensionality (e.g., Linacre, 1998b, 2014c; Smith, 2002; Tennant & Pallant, 2006). One approach is based on examining mean-square infit and outfit statistics. When these statistics are sufficiently close to their expected values, evidence in favor of psychometric unidimensionality is provided. This was the rationale applied to the criterion measurement results discussed in the preceding chapter. Yet, infit and outfit statistics refer to one examinee, rater, or criterion at a time, and thus are more sensitive to detecting local deviations from Rasch model expectations (e.g., due to guessing, response sets, etc.), as compared to the generally more subtle, but pervasive, impact of a secondary dimension (Linacre,

2014c). Furthermore, in case of misfit, it does not follow that the assumption of unidimensionality is to be rejected right away. Data–model misfit can be caused by a host of factors; just one of these factors refers to multidimensionality of the construct being measured.

Another approach is to conduct a *principal component analysis* (PCA) of standardized residuals (Chou & Wang, 2010; Linacre, 1998b, 2014c; Smith, 2002). Considering a two-facet testing situation, where examinees respond to test items, the basic idea of the residual PCA approach is as follows. If the data closely fit the Rasch model, most of the non-random variance found in the data can be accounted for by a single latent dimension. Thus, when the primary measurement dimension (e.g., item difficulty) has been extracted, the proportion of the variance of the residuals should be fairly low, as compared to the proportion of raw-score variance of observations explained by Rasch measures, and the residuals should show no evidence of meaningful structure; that is, the residual factor loadings should be small, random, and not suggestive of a second or even third dimension.

If the analysis yields evidence of a non-negligible proportion of variance in the residuals, and if this variance can be accounted for by a second dimension that is judged to be significant enough to impact the empirical meaning or use of the measures, one may consider taking remedial action such as eliminating items, which are held responsible for introducing another dimension, or grouping the items into subtests and constructing additional latent variables (Linacre, 1998b). Note, however, that in an assessment context comprising more than two facets, the analysis is complicated by the fact that a PCA of residuals requires as input a rectangular data matrix; that is, the many-facet data need to be formatted into a matrix comprising rows and columns. For example, when the rater facet is tested for unidimensionality, each rater is placed in a column of that matrix, and combinations of examinees and criteria are placed in the rows (the FACETS program provides users with a dialog box to accomplish this). Then, unidimensionality can be tested using the PCA subroutine as implemented in the WINSTEPS Rasch measurement program (Linacre, 2014c). Specifically, a PCA of the residuals associated with raters would help to find out whether there are raters who jointly define a second dimension.

Wolfe and McVay (2012) demonstrated the use of a PCA for identifying raters who exhibited a *randomness* (or *inaccuracy*) *effect*; that is, raters who were overly inconsistent in the way they applied one or more rating scales (see Myford & Wolfe, 2004). Drawing on an empirical data set, where 40 raters assigned scores on a four-category rating scale to a common set of 400 student essays (a two-facet situation), Wolfe and McVay were able to classify seven raters as inaccurate because (a) their outfit statistic exceeded the critical value of 1.30, *and* (b) the observed inconsistency was *not* attributable to the influence of a construct-irrelevant, secondary dimension, that is, these raters' loadings on the first principal component of the residuals were less than .40 (absolute value). When, however, the absolute values of the rater loadings were greater than .40, Wolfe and McVay classified the raters as exhibiting a *differential dimensionality effect*.

A related technique, or set of techniques, utilizes procedures for detecting *differential item functioning* (DIF). A study of DIF examines the relationship between examinee responses to items and another variable (the grouping variable; e.g., gender, ethnicity, or first language), conditional on a measure of the intended construct (e.g., reading comprehension in a foreign language). The research question then is whether, after controlling for the construct, the item responses are related to group membership. If so, then DIF is said to be present (e.g., Ferne & Rupp, 2007; Osterlind & Everson, 2009; Smith, 2004a). For example, a reading comprehension item would exhibit DIF related to gender if female examinees answered the item correctly more often than equally proficient male examinees. Put another way, items showing DIF introduce a *construct-irrelevant* dimension into the measurement system. Within many-facet Rasch measurement, the same basic approach can be employed to study differential functioning in any of the facets involved. Section 8.4 provides a detailed discussion of the many-facet extension of DIF analysis.

When there is strong empirical evidence pointing to a multidimensional construct, or when theoretical considerations clearly suggest postulating multiple latent dimensions, unidimensional models may be abandoned in favor of a multidimensional approach. For example, reading comprehension items may demand distinct cognitive operations from examinees to provide the correct answer, with each kind of operation corresponding to a different dimension; or a mathematics test may address multiple domains, including reasoning, problem solving, and spatial skills, with each domain calling for a separate dimension.

The basic assumption underlying the use of *multidimensional* IRT or Rasch models is that examinees vary on a number of different proficiency dimensions. In other words, an examinee's location is a point in a multidimensional space rather than a point along a single latent continuum.

At first sight, multidimensional models appear attractive because they allow for different competency profiles, cognitive components, or learning styles, but they complicate the assignment of levels because decisions must be made (explicitly or implicitly) about the degree to which strengths along one dimension compensate for weaknesses along another dimension. In practice, the levels are defined along one dimension, and so the reported results must also lie along that one dimension.

It should also be noted that some multidimensional IRT models can produce paradoxical results; that is, getting an item correct may actually *decrease* the estimate of an examinee's proficiency in some dimension (Hooker, Finkelman, & Schwartzman, 2009). Surely, this calls into question the appropriateness of such models for assigning scores or levels to examinees, particularly in high-stakes testing.

Until recently, multidimensional IRT modeling approaches have only rarely been adopted in educational or language testing contexts (for some illustrative applications, see Hartig & Höhler, 2008; Liu, Wilson, & Paek, 2008). General reviews have been provided by Briggs and Wilson (2004), Carstensen and Rost (2007), Reckase (2009), and Reise, Cook, and Moore (2015). The FACETS program, which is used throughout the sample data analysis in this book, exclusively implements unidimensional Rasch models.

8.3 Partial credit and hybrid models

When the observations refer to polytomous responses, the implied structure of the response scale needs to be examined. The facets model used in the previous analysis was based on the assumption that all three criteria shared a *common* rating scale structure. That is, each category on one criterion scale (e.g., *TDN 3* on *global impression*) was assumed to be functionally equivalent to the same category on the other criterion scales (i.e., *TDN 3* on *task fulfillment* and on *linguistic realization*). Therefore, the MFRM analysis yielded only a single measurement table containing the rating scale category statistics (Table 7.3), and it yielded only a single set of category probability curves (Figure 7.3). The category statistics provided a summary of how the raters (as a group) used each of the four categories across the three criterion scales. Put differently, the category thresholds were assumed to be constant across the criteria.

To investigate the extent to which this assumption was actually borne out in the data, the model statement shown in Equation 2.11 was modified by changing the specification of the category coefficient term from τ_k (with a single index) to τ_{ik} (with a double index). The revised model statement would be specified as follows:

$$\ln\left[\frac{p_{nijk}}{p_{nijk-1}}\right] = \theta_n - \beta_i - \alpha_j - \tau_{ik}, \tag{8.1}$$

where all the parameters are as in Equation 2.11 except for the τ_{ik} term, which now represents the difficulty of scale category k relative to scale category $k - 1$ on criterion i.

Equation 8.1 is an expression for a *criterion-related three-facet partial credit model*. This model could also be called a *hybrid model*, since it combines a partial-credit component applied to the criteria with a rating scale component applied to the raters (Myford & Wolfe, 2003). In the FACETS specification file (Table 4.1), this model can be requested using the command "Model=?,?,#,R5" instead of "Model=?,?,?,R5".

More specifically, the τ_{ik} term indicates that the rating scale for each criterion is modeled to have its own category structure; that is, the structure of the rating scale is allowed to vary from one criterion to another. For example, a rating of *TDN 4* on *global impression* may be more difficult (or easier) for examinees to attain relative to *TDN 5* than is a rating of *TDN 4* on *task fulfillment*. A criterion-related partial credit MFRM analysis reveals the scale structure of each individual criterion scale and thus provides information about how the group of raters used each category on each criterion.

Figure 8.1 shows the Wright map resulting from the partial credit analysis of the sample data based on the model presented in Equation 8.1. The headings of the first four columns are the same as before (see Figure 4.1), with only slight changes in the estimates of parameters for examinees, raters, and criteria. But now each criterion has its own rating scale structure.

Fig. 8.1: Wright map from the many-facet partial credit analysis. Each star in the second column represents three examinees, and a dot represents one or two examinees. LR = linguistic realization. TF = task fulfillment. GI = global impression. The horizontal dashed lines in the last three columns indicate the category threshold measures for each of the three criterion scales.

Logit	**Examinees**	**Raters**	**Criteria**	**Rating scale for each criterion**		
	High	*Severe*	*Difficult*	GI	TF	LR
				(TDN 5)	(TDN 5)	(TDN 5)
	.					
7						
	.					
6	*.					
	*.					
	*.					
5	*.					
	**					
4	***.					
	**.			-----	-----	-----
	**.					
3	**.					
	***					
	**.	16				
2	*******.	13 14				TDN 4
	***.			TDN 4	TDN 4	
	***.	09 15				
1	*****	05				
	***.					
	****.	04	LR TF			
0	***	06 08 11 18		-----	-----	-----
	******					
	****.	17				
-1	***.	10 12	GI			
	**	02				
	*****					
-2	**	03		TDN 3	TDN 3	TDN 3
	**.	01 07				
	**.					
-3	**.					
	*					
	***.			-----	-----	
-4	.					-----
	.					
	.					
-5	*					
	.					
	.					
-6	.					
	.					
	Low	*Lenient*	*Easy*	(below 3)	(below 3)	(below 3)

Table 8.1: Rating Scale Category Calibrations for Each Criterion.

	Global impression		**Task fulfillment**		**Linguistic realization**		**Threshold**	
Category	**Threshold**	***SE***	**Threshold**	***SE***	**Threshold**	***SE***	***M***	***SD***
TDN 3	−3.48	0.22	−3.50	0.17	−3.78	0.18	−3.59	0.17
TDN 4	−0.20	0.14	−0.20	0.13	0.05	0.13	−0.12	0.14
TDN 5	3.68	0.13	3.70	0.15	3.73	0.16	3.70	0.03

Note. Thresholds are Rasch-Andrich thresholds.

The corresponding criterion scales are shown in the last three columns (in the order the scales were entered into FACETS).

Particularly interesting are the locations of the criterion-specific category thresholds, indicated by horizontal dashed lines. Regarding *global impression* and *task fulfillment*, differences between threshold locations were negligibly small. Only the location of the threshold between categories *below TDN 3* and *TDN 3* of *linguistic realization* was placed slightly lower, as compared to the other two scales. Thus, as a group, raters used the TDN scale in much the same way across the three criteria.

Table 8.1 summarizes the rating scale category calibrations (i.e., Rasch-Andrich thresholds) for each criterion, as well as the means and standard deviations of these threshold estimates. The results confirm that the category calibrations were highly consistent across criteria. In each case, the differences between mean thresholds of rating scale categories were substantially larger than the corresponding standard deviations (see the last two columns of Table 8.1). In addition, the thresholds for each criterion were widely separated along the examinee proficiency scale. Thus, on each criterion, examinees had a high probability of being correctly classified into a rating scale category that best described their proficiency. In other words, the three criteria discriminated equally well between high- and low-proficiency examinees.[10]

Two other kinds of hybrid models, presented only briefly here, result from further varying the specification of the category coefficient. The first model is suited to studying the way in which *each* rater used the set of criterion scales:

10 On the basis of the criterion-related partial credit model, the average threshold difference computed for a particular criterion can be used as an *indirect* measure of the criterion's discrimination. To estimate the discrimination (or slope) parameter directly, the *generalized partial credit model* (Muraki, 1992) or the *generalized multilevel facets model* (Wang & Liu, 2007) could be employed (see also Embretson & Reise, 2000; Linacre, 2006b; Rost, 2004).

$$\ln\left[\frac{p_{nijk}}{p_{nijk-1}}\right] = \theta_n - \beta_i - \alpha_j - \tau_{jk}. \tag{8.2}$$

The only difference from Equation 8.1 is that the τ_{jk} term now represents the difficulty of scale category k relative to scale category $k - 1$ for rater j.

Equation 8.2 is an expression for a *rater-related three-facet partial credit model.* This model combines a partial-credit component applied to the raters with a rating scale component applied to the criteria (Myford & Wolfe, 2003; see also Congdon & McQueen, 2000b; Wolfe, 2009). More specifically, the τ_{jk} term indicates that the rating scale for each rater is modeled to have its own category structure; that is, the structure of the rating scale is allowed to vary from one rater to another. A rater-related partial credit MFRM analysis reveals the pattern that individual raters exhibited when using the set of three criterion scales. In other words, this analysis would show how a particular rater used each category of the rating scale *across all* criteria. Section 5.2 contained an illustrative application of the model within the context of identifying central tendency effects. That model can be requested in the FACETS specification file by inserting the command "Model=?,#,?,R5" (see Table 4.1).

Finally, to look at the way *each* rater used each category of the rating scale on *each* criterion, the partial-credit components from the models specified in Equations 8.1 and 8.2 would have to be merged:

$$\ln\left[\frac{p_{nijk}}{p_{nijk-1}}\right] = \theta_n - \beta_i - \alpha_j - \tau_{ijk}. \tag{8.3}$$

Now the τ_{ijk} term (note the triple index) represents the difficulty of scale category k relative to scale category $k - 1$ for criterion i and rater j.

Equation 8.3 is an expression for a *criterion- and rater-related three-facet partial credit model.* This model combines a partial-credit component applied to the criteria with a partial-credit component applied to the raters (Myford & Wolfe, 2003). More specifically, the τ_{ijk} term indicates that the rating scale for each criterion *and* each rater is modeled to have its own category structure. A combined criterion- and rater-related partial credit MFRM analysis reveals the pattern that individual raters exhibited when using each of the criterion scales. The corresponding command in the FACETS specification file would be "Model=?,#,#,R5" (see Table 4.1).

Compared to their rating scale counterparts, partial credit model variants generally require larger sample sizes in order to achieve similar stability of parameter estimates across samples. According to Linacre (1994, 2004b, 2014b; see also Table 7.2), estimates with some degree of stability across samples may be obtained when there are at least 30 observations per element, and at least 10 observations per rating scale category. Thus, when a model such as the one specified in Equation 8.3 were to be used, the minimum requirement of 10 observations per category would be much harder to satisfy than when the rating scale model of Equation 4.1 were chosen. This is because, in the partial credit model, category coefficients would have to be estimated for each criterion–rater combination separately.

8.4 Modeling facet interactions

The MFRM models discussed so far allow the researcher to single out the effect that each facet has on the measurement results. Yet, these models were not designed to take possible interactions between facets into account. That is why they are also called *main-effects models* (e.g., Rost & Walter, 2006; Schumacker, 1996; Schumacker & Lunz, 1997). As mentioned in the discussion of the conceptual–psychometric framework (Section 3.3), interactions between facets may come into play and, thus, are an issue when modeling performance assessments.

Based on parameter estimates for examinees, raters, criteria, etc., various interactions between facets, or differential facet functioning (DFF), can be examined. When referring to interactions involving raters, for example, interactions between raters and examinee gender groups, an interaction analysis is said to address *differential rater functioning* (DRF) or *rater bias* (e.g., Bachman, 2004; Du et al., 1996; Engelhard, 2007a; McNamara, 1996; Myford & Wolfe, 2003). Rater bias threatens the *fairness* of an assessment, which may be defined as "comparable validity for *identifiable* and *relevant* groups across all stages of assessment" (Xi, 2010, p. 154). Depending on the number of facets considered, the analysis may address two-way interactions, three-way interactions, or even higher-way interactions.

Regarding the purpose of a many-facet interaction analysis, it is useful to distinguish between exploratory and confirmatory approaches. To begin with, an *exploratory* interaction analysis aims at identifying systematic deviations from model expectations without any specific hypothesis in mind. That is, each and every combination of elements from two or more different facets is scanned for significant differences between observed and expected scores. The expected scores are derived from the basic MFRM model that does not include any interaction, that is, from the main-effects model. Significant differences are flagged and then inspected more closely. Possibly, some kind of post-hoc explanation can be reached that may in turn serve to devise a more focused interaction analysis.

Based on a theoretical rationale, on prior research, or on systematic observations, a researcher may want to test a specific interaction hypothesis; that is, a hypothesis that explicitly states which facets or which subgroups of elements of particular facets are likely to be involved in generating patterns of systematic violations of model expectations. In this kind of situation, a *confirmatory* interaction analysis is called for. Typically, in a confirmatory analysis some distal variable such as examinee gender or time of scoring session is considered a facet potentially exerting additional influence on the ratings.

8.4.1 Exploratory interaction analysis

To conduct an exploratory interaction analysis, the basic MFRM model is extended by adding a separate parameter that represents the interaction between the relevant facets. For example, considering again the model specified in Equation 2.11, the interaction between the examinee facet and the rater facet can be studied by adding an Examinee-by-Rater interaction parameter. The model statement then becomes:

$$\ln\left[\frac{p_{nijk}}{p_{nijk-1}}\right] = \theta_n - \beta_i - \alpha_j - \varphi_{nj} - \tau_k, \qquad (8.4)$$

where φ_{nj} is the Examinee-by-Rater interaction parameter, also called *bias parameter* (or *bias term*).

In the FACETS specification file (see Table 4.1), this model is requested by changing the model definition from "Model = ?,?,?,R5" to "Model = ?B,?B,?,R5". The elements of each facet marked by "B" are subjected to the interaction analysis. Of course, at least two "B" terms are required.

FACETS reports a *bias statistic*, which can be used to judge the statistical significance of the size of the bias parameter estimate. That is, this statistic provides a test of the hypothesis that there is no bias apart from measurement error. The bias statistic is approximately distributed as a *t* statistic (with *df* = number of observations – 1). Referring to the bias term specified in Equation 8.4, the bias statistic is

$$t_{nj} = \hat{\varphi}_{nj} / SE_{nj}, \qquad (8.5)$$

where SE_{nj} is the standard error of the bias parameter estimate.

An Examinee-by-Rater interaction analysis is suited to investigate whether each rater maintained a uniform level of severity across examinees or whether particular raters scored some examinees' performance more harshly or leniently than expected. Another two-way interaction analysis would test for patterns of unexpected ratings related to particular scoring criteria. To examine whether the combination of a particular rater and a particular criterion resulted in too harsh or too lenient scores awarded to some examinees, a three-way interaction analysis could be performed.

Drawing again on the essay rating data, Table 8.2 presents summary statistics showing the group-level results for these three bias analyses, that is, for the two two-way analyses (Examinee-by-Rater, Criterion-by-Rater) and for the three-way analysis (Examinee-by-Criterion-by-Rater).

The table lists the total number of combinations of facet elements considered in each interaction analysis (i.e., excluding elements with extreme scores), the percentage of (absolute) t values equal or greater than 2, the percentage of statistically significant t values, the minimum and maximum t values (along with their degrees of freedom), as well as the means and standard deviations of the respective t values.

The percentage values for the Examinee-by-Rater and the Examinee-by-Criterion-by-Rater interactions were negligibly low. However, a considerable number of combinations of raters and criteria were associated with substantial differences between observed and expected scores; there were 10 large t values, of which 8 (14.81%) were statistically significant. This indicates that some raters failed to keep their level of severity across the three criteria. They tended instead to alternate between harsher ratings on one criterion and more lenient ratings on another criterion.

The criterion-related fluctuations in rater bias are displayed in Figure 8.2. For each Criterion-by-Rater combination, the value of the bias statistic t is shown along the vertical axis. Values of t greater than 0 indicate observed scores that are higher than expected based on the model (i.e., a tendency toward leniency), and values of t smaller than 0 indicate observed scores that are lower than expected (i.e., a tendency toward severity). For ease of interpretation, the figure includes the upper and lower quality control limits and shows which t values were statistically significant at the .05 level.

Table 8.2: Summary Statistics for the Exploratory Interaction Analysis.

Statistic	Examinee × Rater	Criterion × Rater	Examinee × Criterion × Rater
N	611	54	1833
% large *t*-values[a]	3.93	18.52	1.42
% sign. *t*-values[b]	0.00	14.81	0.00
Min-*t* (*df*)	−3.51 (2)	−2.71* (19)	−2.72 (1)
Max-*t* (*df*)	3.30 (2)	2.78* (24)	2.56 (1)
M	−0.02	0.00	−0.05
SD	0.92	1.31	0.77

Note. N = number of element combinations. [a]Percentage of absolute t-values equal or greater than 2.00. [b]Percentage of t-values statistically significant at $p < .05$. * $p < .05$.

As can be seen, Rater 02 exhibited a significant leniency bias toward *global impression* and tended to award unduly severe ratings on *task fulfillment*. Rater 18 exhibited a strong severity bias toward *task fulfillment*, whereas his or her ratings on *global impression* and *linguistic realization* were within control limits.

Altogether there were five raters showing at least one significant criterion-related bias. Four biases were in the direction of severity; the other four indicated the presence of a pronounced tendency toward leniency. Note also that one rater (i.e., Rater 11) tended to assign highly similar ratings across the three criteria, though, as shown in Table 7.1, *linguistic realization* and *task fulfillment* proved to be more difficult than *global impression*. Hence, it may well be that Rater 11 exhibited a halo effect, showing less discrimination among criteria than warranted by the differences in criterion difficulty measures (see Section 5.2).

Graphical displays of rater bias of the kind illustrated in Figure 8.2 are called *bias control charts* or *bias diagrams*. Bias diagrams are a very useful component of rater monitoring and/or rater training activities targeted at diminishing unwanted variability in rater behavior (e.g., Engelhard, 2002; McNamara, 1996; Stahl & Lunz, 1996).

Fig. 8.2: Bias diagram showing the interaction between raters and criteria (GI = global impression, TF = task fulfillment, LR = linguistic realization). Also shown are upper and lower quality control limits (horizontal dashed lines placed at 2.0 and –2.0, respectively). Statistically significant t-values are circled.

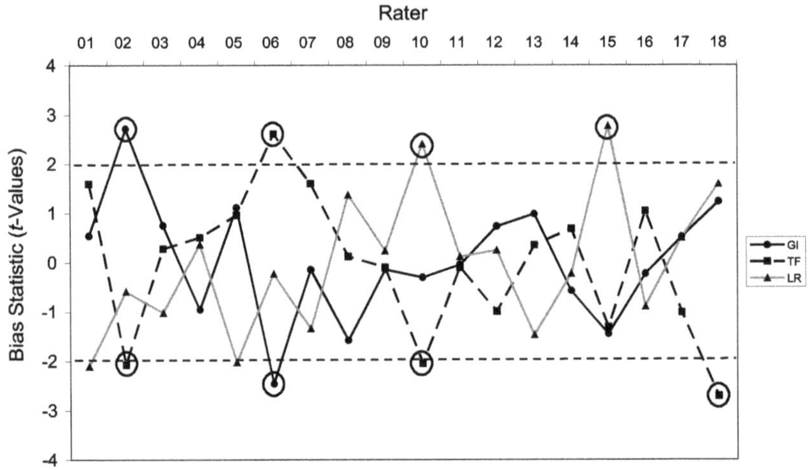

At the individual level, that is, at the level of each individual rater, bias diagrams may be supplemented with *bias control tables*. These tables typically contain more detailed statistical information on possible rater bias. Table 8.3 depicts the criterion-related bias control findings for Rater 05 excerpted from the FACETS output. The severity estimate for this rater was 1.05 logits (*SE* = 0.19; see Table 5.1).

For each criterion, the table lists the difficulty measure, the number of ratings that went into the bias estimation, the observed score (i.e., the sum of the TDNs across examinees), the expected score (based on the parameter estimates), and the average difference between the observed score and the expected score. The last four columns are particularly relevant for an evaluation of potential rater bias related to criteria. Thus, the "Bias Measure" column gives the estimate of the interaction parameter for Rater 05 and each criterion (i.e., the bias in terms of the logit scale). Bias estimates greater than 0 indicate observed scores that are higher than expected based on the model, while estimates smaller than 0 indicate observed scores that are lower than expected. Dividing the bias measure by its standard error yields the value of the bias statistic *t*. The probability associated with each *t* value is given in the last column.

As already shown in Figure 8.2, the probability column reveals that one of the bias statistics approached the conventional .05 significance level. Thus, the bias measure related to *linguistic realization* reflects an observed score much smaller than expected. Summed over the 39 examinees receiving non-extreme scores, the observed score is about 6 scale points smaller than the expected score, giving an average observed–expected difference of –0.16. The bias estimate is –0.68 logits (*SE* = 0.34). Since the overall difficulty measure of this criterion is 0.53 logits, the difficulty of *linguistic realization* as specifically related to Rater 05 is 1.21 logits (i.e., 0.53 logits – [–0.68 logits]). In other words, this criterion's *local difficulty* is 1.21 logits; alternatively, one could say that this rater's *local severity* is 1.73 logits (i.e., 1.05 logits – [–0.68 logits]).

Table 8.3: Results from the Criterion-by-Rater Bias Analysis for Rater 05.

Criterion	Difficulty Measure	*N* of Ratings	Obs. Score	Exp. Score	Obs. – expected (*M*)	Bias Measure	*SE*	*t*	*p*
LR	0.53	39	117	123.2	–0.16	–0.68	0.34	–2.02	.0503
TF	0.43	39	127	124.1	0.07	0.31	0.33	0.96	.3449
GI	–0.97	39	141	137.5	0.09	0.36	0.32	1.11	.2730

Note. LR = linguistic realization. TF = task fulfillment. GI = global impression. *t* = bias statistic.

Table 8.4: Selected Results from the Examinee-by-Rater Bias Analysis for Rater 05.

Examinee	Proficiency Measure	*N* of Ratings	Obs. Score	Exp. Score	Obs. – expected (*M*)	Bias Measure	*SE*	*t*	*p*
012	3.59	3	13	12.5	0.15	0.61	1.15	0.53	.6503
284	0.01	3	9	9.7	–0.23	–0.83	1.11	–0.75	.5318
133	–0.21	3	8	9.5	–0.50	–1.82	1.10	–1.65	.2414
295	–0.73	3	12	9.1	0.98	3.57	1.16	3.08	.0914
251	–3.79	3	6	6.8	–0.25	–0.75	1.70	–0.44	.7001

Note. LR = linguistic realization. TF = task fulfillment. GI = global impression. *t* = bias statistic.

Basically the same kind of table can be constructed with regard to the inspection of possible rater bias related to examinees. Table 8.4 presents selected results of the examinee-related bias analysis for Rater 05.

For each examinee, Table 8.4 lists the proficiency measure, the number of ratings (one rating for each criterion), the observed score (i.e., the sum of the TDNs awarded to the examinee across criteria), the expected score (based on the parameter estimates), and the average difference between the observed score and the expected score. As before, bias estimates greater than 0 indicate observed scores that are higher than expected based on the model, while estimates smaller than 0 indicate observed scores that are lower than expected.

As judged by their associated probabilities, none of the bias statistics reached the .05 level of significance. Yet, statistical significance critically hinges on the number of observations, which in the present case was very small. Hence, as mentioned above, it is reasonable to consider *t*'s with an absolute value of at least 2 as indicative of substantial rater bias. Following this guideline, there is one bias measure that reflected an observed score much higher than expected (marginally significant at the .10 level): the bias measure for Examinee 295.

Summed over the three criterion ratings, this examinee's observed score is almost 3 scale points higher than the expected score, resulting in an average observed–expected difference of 0.98. The bias estimate is 3.57 logits ($SE = 1.16$), which means that, from Rater's 05 perspective, Examinee 295 is 3.57 logits more proficient than his or her overall measure. Hence, the examinee's proficiency, as specifically viewed by Rater 05, is as high as 2.84 logits (i.e., –0.73 logits + 3.57 logits). Put differently, Examinee 295 has a *local proficiency* of 2.84 logits; or, given that an examinee's proficiency is a relatively stable characteristic, it generally makes more sense to say that Rater 05 has a *local severity* of –2.52 logits (i.e., 1.05 logits – 3.57 logits); thus, this rater is markedly lenient when it comes to rating Examinee 295. Note that higher examinee proficiency measures refer to *higher* observed scores, whereas higher rater severity (and higher criterion difficulty) measures refer to *lower* observed scores. That is why the bias estimate is added to the logit value in the case of examinees, but subtracted from the logit value in the case of raters (and criteria).

FACETS bias analysis output also shows direct comparisons or contrasts between two elements of the same facet. For example, Rater 05 (the "target") is 3.57 logits more lenient when rating Examinee 295, but 1.82 logits less lenient when rating Examinee 133. Combining these two biases leads to the conclusion that Rater 05 is 5.39 logits more lenient with Examinee 295 than with Examinee 133. In FACETS output, the bias difference is called *target contrast*. Using a paired *t* test, this contrast is shown to be statistically significant, $t(3) = 3.37, p < .05$.

Fig. 8.3: Bias diagram for Rater 05. Dots represent examinees with proficiency measures along the horizontal axis and the associated values of the bias statistic along the vertical axis. Also shown are upper and lower quality control limits (dashed lines placed at 2.0 and –2.0, respectively).

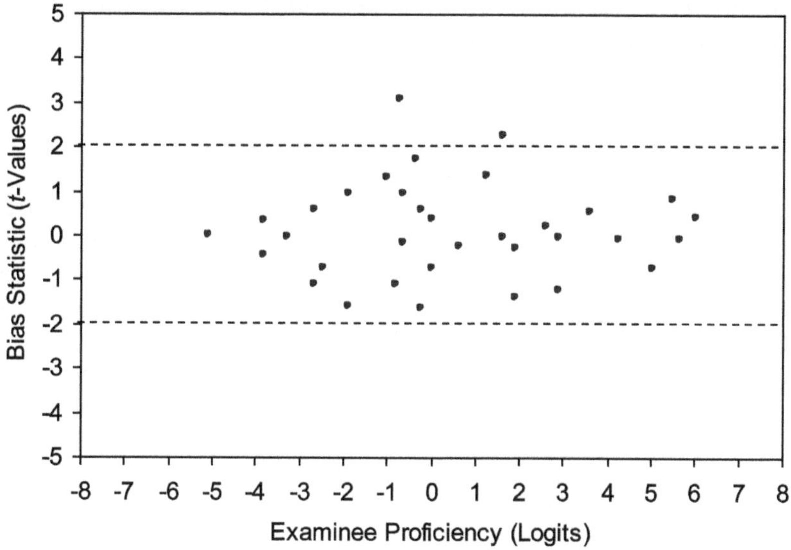

The complete distribution of *t* values for Rater 05 plotted against the proficiency measures of the examinees scored by this rater is displayed in Figure 8.3.[11] Again, the upper and lower quality control limits are shown. As can be seen, only two bias statistic values fell outside these limits; one of these values belonged to the case of Examinee 295 discussed above. Since the horizontal axis refers to the examinee proficiency measures, a rough visual test can be made of whether Rater 05's bias tendency was correlated with the proficiency of the examinees he or she rated. Here, as with all the other raters studied, no such tendency was evident (Pearson's *r* for the data depicted in Figure 8.3 was .06, *ns*).

11 Figure 8.3 shows 34 dots, of which 5 dots are duplicates due to identical value pairs; dots for 2 examinees are missing because of extreme scores awarded by all raters involved.

8.4.2 Confirmatory interaction analysis

To conduct a confirmatory interaction analysis, the basic model specification is expanded by adding at least two parameters, a new facet parameter and an interaction parameter. In this case, the first added parameter represents the facet that is the focus of the hypothesis; the second added parameter represents the interaction between that facet and some other facet already included in the model.

Hitherto, the bulk of research adopting a confirmatory approach concerned the rater facet, that is, differential rater functioning (DRF). In particular, researchers have looked at DRF related to examinee gender (e.g., Du & Wright, 1997; Eckes, 2005b; Engelhard & Myford, 2003) or DRF over time (also called *rater drift*; e.g., Congdon & McQueen, 2000a; Hoskens & Wilson, 2001; Lamprianou, 2006; Lim, 2011; Lunz, Stahl, & Wright, 1996; O'Neill & Lunz, 2000; Wilson & Case, 2000; Wolfe, Moulder, & Myford, 2001).

In a study of rater drift, *time of rating* would be considered a relevant facet. Adding a time facet to the basic model equation would allow the mean of the ratings to vary across time, but the severity of each individual rater would still be modeled as static. In order to identify individual raters who *change* their levels of severity over time, a parameter representing the interaction between the time facet and the rater facet would have to be added to the model. Changes in rating behavior that are dependent on the time of rating may manifest themselves not only in variations of rater severity, but also in variations of rater accuracy, or in variations of scale category usage (for a detailed discussion, see Myford & Wolfe, 2009; Wolfe et al., 2007).

Next, the basic procedure of a confirmatory interaction analysis is demonstrated, focusing on the analysis of DRF related to examinee gender (see also Eckes, 2005b; Engelhard & Myford, 2003).[12] The research question was: Did any of the raters show evidence of differential severity/leniency, rating female exami-

12 Two pieces of hidden information might have contributed to gender bias in the sample data: (a) each essay as well as each scoring sheet had a label attached to it, which contained, in addition to an identification number and other technical details, the examinee's full name (following the implementation of automated scanning procedures this early practice has been changed to examinee identification by number only); (b) there is some empirical evidence that raters are able to identify the gender of examinees based on handwriting alone (Boulet & McKinley, 2005; Emerling, 1991; see also Haswell & Haswell, 1996).

nees' essays (or male examinees' essays) more severely or leniently than expected or was the ordering of raters by severity invariant across gender groups?

To answer this question, two terms were added to the model in Equation 2.11: (a) a facet term representing the examinee gender group, and (b) an interaction term representing the Rater-by-Gender Group interaction parameter. Thus, the modified model that was to provide a test of the gender bias hypothesis looked like this:

$$\ln\left[\frac{p_{nijk}}{p_{nijk-1}}\right] = \theta_n - \beta_i - \alpha_j - \gamma_g - \varphi_{jg} - \tau_k, \qquad (8.6)$$

where p_{nijk} is the probability of examinee n of gender group g receiving a rating of k on criterion i from rater j, p_{nijk-1} is the probability of examinee n of gender group g receiving a rating of $k - 1$ on criterion i from rater j, γ_g is the gender facet term, and ϕ_{jg} is the Rater-by-Gender Group interaction term; all other terms are as in Equation 2.11.

In the present example, the gender bias analysis was performed by estimating proficiency measures for each group of female and male examinees along with differential proficiency measures for each and every combination of an individual rater with the respective gender group. Specifically, in order to compute the Rater-by-Gender Group interaction term, a two-step calibration was used (see Myford & Wolfe, 2003). In Step I, all parameters except ϕ_{jg} were estimated. In Step II, all parameters except ϕ_{jg} were anchored to the values estimated during the first step; then, parameter estimates and standard errors for ϕ_{jg} were obtained.

The new input data file "W002G.txt" contained the gender label (male = "1", female = "2") in the fourth column (right after the three-digit examinee label). In terms of the FACETS specification file (see Table 4.1), the model definition for the Step I analysis was changed to "Model=?,?,?,?,R5". Note that the model definition now specifies four facets: examinees, examinee gender, raters, and criteria.

To create the anchor output file, the command "Output=W002G.out, W002G.anc" was inserted into the specifications; the first of these output files will contain the main results of the Step I analysis, and the second output file will contain the specifications along with the anchoring values to be used in Step II. Changing the model definition in this anchor file to "Model=?,?B,?B,?" (i.e., interaction between examinee gender and raters) and then running that file, the gender bias analysis will be performed.

The null hypothesis that there is no gender bias (i.e., $\phi_{jg} = 0$) is tested by means of the t statistic introduced earlier:

$$t_{jg} = \hat{\varphi}_{jg} / SE_{jg}, \tag{8.7}$$

where SE_{jg} is the standard error of the gender bias parameter estimate.

A statistically significant interaction term would provide evidence for DRF. When DRF occurs, the particular Rater-by-Gender Group combination results in unexpectedly low or unexpectedly high ratings, given the rater's level of severity and the gender group's level of proficiency.

At the *group level*, three statistical indicators may provide information on gender bias (Myford & Wolfe, 2004): (a) the fixed chi-square statistic, to find out whether female and male examinees shared the same calibrated level of performance, (b) the gender separation index, to determine the number of statistically distinct levels of performance among the gender groups, and (c) the reliability of gender separation, to see how well female and male examinees were separated in terms of their performances.

However, as Myford and Wolfe (2004) noted, the information provided by each of these summary statistics may be interpreted as demonstrating group-level rater differential severity/leniency only if the researcher has *prior* knowledge about whether the average measures of the gender groups should differ. Since gender differences in verbal ability have been extensively studied, though in different contexts and using different methodological approaches, knowledge on this issue was available (e.g., Cole, 1997; Du & Wright 1997; Engelhard, Gordon, & Gabrielson, 1991; Hedges & Nowell, 1995; Hyde & Linn, 1988; Mattern, Camara, & Kobrin, 2007). For instance, in a meta-analysis covering 165 studies, Hyde and Linn (1988) found an overall mean effect size of 0.11, indicating a slight female superiority in verbal performance. More specific analyses revealed that the mean effect size was 0.09 ($p < .05$) for essay writing, and 0.33 ($p < .05$) for speech production.[13] Thus, the expectation in the present study was that females would outperform males in the writing section, albeit only to a small degree.

Evidence of gender bias, therefore, would require that the measures for the gender facet either were very small (and not significantly different), indicating gender bias favoring males, or very large (and significantly different), indicating gender bias favoring females.

13 The effect size computed for each study was defined as the mean for females minus the mean for males, divided by the pooled within-gender standard deviation (see Hedges & Olkin, 1985).

The analysis revealed that the proficiency measure for females was 0.33 logits (SE = 0.07) and that for males was –0.33 logits (SE = 0.07). This logit difference was statistically significant: homogeneity statistic Q_g (1) = 47.8 ($p < .01$). Similarly, the gender separation index was 6.71, and the reliability of gender separation was .96.

Therefore, it seems safe to conclude that females performed significantly better than males, a conclusion that is in line with expectations based on prior research (see, for highly congruent findings in a large-scale writing assessment context, Du & Wright, 1997; Gyagenda & Engelhard, 2009). Thus, there was no evidence of a group-level differential severity/leniency effect.

Deeper insight into the gender bias issue may be gained through an *individual-level* analysis. An analysis at this level indicates whether there were individual raters that displayed differential severity in their ratings.

FACETS provided two kinds of relevant evidence, each referring to the same underlying bias/interaction information, yet from different perspectives. First, each rater was crossed with each gender group to pinpoint ratings that were highly unexpected given the pattern revealed in the overall analysis. As discussed above, any significant bias found here would provide evidence of differential rater functioning. Second, the severity of a particular rater when rating females was compared to this rater's severity when rating males. In each perspective, significant t values would provide evidence of gender bias.

Given the results of the present group-level analysis, it was not surprising that the analysis failed to find any evidence of individual-level bias, no matter which perspective was taken. In the first (crossed) perspective, t values ranged from –0.81 to 0.91; in the second (pairwise) perspective t values ranged from –1.21 to 1.17 (all t's non-significant). Nonetheless, for the purposes of illustration, Table 8.5 presents selected findings from the crossed individual-level analysis.

Table 8.5: Selected Results from the Individual-Level Gender-Bias Analysis.

Rater	Severity Measure	Exam. Gender	*N* of Ratings	Obs. Score	Exp. Score	Obs. – exp. (*M*)	Bias Measure	*SE*	*t*	*p*
05	1.04	Female	54	202	199.5	0.05	0.19	0.28	0.70	.4851
		Male	69	213	214.8	–0.03	–0.12	0.25	–0.46	.6502
11	0.14	Female	24	95	92.8	0.09	0.37	0.42	0.89	.3805
		Male	33	107	109.2	–0.07	–0.25	0.34	–0.75	.4570
07	–2.24	Female	111	469	472.8	–0.03	–0.17	0.21	–0.80	.4256
		Male	93	360	355.6	0.05	0.19	0.21	0.91	.3644

Note. t = bias statistic.

Fig. 8.4: Gender bias diagram showing the interaction between raters and examinee gender groups.

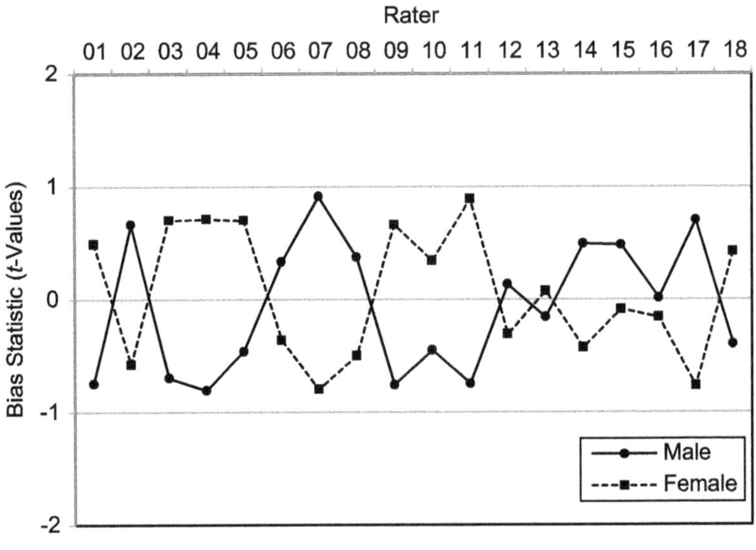

The structure of Table 8.5 is similar to that of Table 8.4, except for the added Examinee Gender column. A positive sign of the bias measure indicates that a particular rater on average awarded to a given gender group higher scores than expected on the basis of the model. Conversely, a negative sign of the bias measure indicates that a particular rater on average awarded to a given gender group lower scores than expected. For example, Rater 05 rated female examinees' performance slightly higher than expected and male examinees' performance slightly lower than expected; Rater 07 showed the opposite rating tendency.

When *multiple* comparisons of raters are made (as in the crossed analysis presented here) critical significance levels should be adjusted to guard against falsely rejecting the null hypothesis that no biases were present (e.g., Engelhard, 2002). To this purpose, methods such as those based on the Bonferroni inequality (see Linacre, 2010b; Myers et al., 2010) or the Benjamini–Hochberg procedure (see Thissen, Steinberg, & Kuang, 2002; Wolfe et al., 2006) can be used.

Figure 8.4 shows the gender bias diagram for the complete set of raters. There are some noticeable differences in gender bias across raters. For example, Rater 07 scored males higher and females lower than expected, whereas Rater 11 exhibited the opposite tendency (see also Table 8.5). Yet, none of the *t* values comes close to the upper and lower quality control limits (at 2.0 and –2.0, respectively). This indicates that none of the differential scoring tendencies reached the level of significance, as the crossed analysis had already shown. Note also that, across raters, there is no consistent tendency to award higher scores than expected to one of the gender groups.

Finally, there is an efficient alternative to the two-step gender bias analysis outlined above. This approach rests on the definition of gender as a *dummy facet* (Linacre, 2002a, 2014b). Specifically, dummy facets are facets that are hypothesized to cause interactions with other facets. Therefore, dummy facets are usually introduced in a measurement design for the sole purpose of studying interactions, not for measuring main effects. Most often dummy facets refer to demographic or other categorical variables describing examinees, raters, or the assessment situation. In terms of the conceptual–psychometric framework discussed in Section 3.3, dummy facets coincide with distal facets.

Thus, if we were *not* interested in main effects of examinee gender, but solely in possible interactions between examinee gender and raters, we could run a bias analysis with gender as a dummy facet. Such an analysis would be easier to perform than the somewhat cumbersome two-step procedure. An excerpt from the FACETS specification file used for the gender bias analysis, including examinee gender as a dummy facet, is shown in Table 8.6.

As described above, there are four facets, and the model definition specifies that we want to study the interaction between examinee gender (Facet 2) and raters (Facet 3). Now, in the facet labels section, examinee gender is defined as Facet 2, a dummy facet, denoted by "D". The "D" has the effect of anchoring all the elements of the dummy facet at 0 logits. Thus, no measures will be estimated for these elements, but they will be included for fit statistics and bias analysis.

Remember that the input data file contained the examinee gender label in the fourth column (directly following the examinee label). When the labels for dummy facet elements are already included in the labels for examinees, FACETS provides a convenient approach to pick out these labels.

Table 8.6: Excerpt from the FACETS Specification File for the Gender Bias Analysis (Defining Examinee Gender as a Dummy Facet).

Specification	Explanation
Title = Essay rating	Title of the MFRM analysis.
Facets = 4	The number of facets is increased from 3 to 4.
Data file = W002G.txt	The input data with an added column for examinee gender.
Model = ?,?B,?B,?,R5	In the model definition, an interaction is specified between Facet 2 (gender) and Facet 3 (raters).
*	End of model definition.
...	(Further specifications as in Table 4.1)
Labels =	The list of labels (identifiers) follows:
1,Examinee	Facet 1, the examinee facet.
1=001	001 is the label of the first examinee.
...	(Examinees 002 to 306 to follow here.)
307=307	307 is the label of the last examinee.
*	End of Facet 1.
2,Gender,D	Facet 2, the gender facet (dummy facet).
1=male	1 is the label of male examinees.
2=female	2 is the label of female examinees.
*	End of Facet 2.
3,Rater	Facet 3, the rater facet.
1=01	01 is the label of the first rater.
...	(Raters 02 to 17 to follow here.)
18=18	18 is the label of the last rater.
*	End of Facet 3.
4,Criterion	Facet 4, the criterion facet.
1=GI	GI is the label of the first criterion, global impression.
2=TF	TF is the label of the second criterion, task fulfillment.
3=LR	LR is the label of the third criterion, linguistic realization.
*	End of Facet 4.

For example, let the label for the first (male) examinee be "0011", with the fourth (appended) digit coding this examinee's gender; that is, the corresponding line in the specification file would read "1=0011". Given this examinee label definition, the following statement would tell FACETS to get the gender information directly from the examinee label and to use it in the analysis: "Dvalue=2,1,4,1". FACETS decodes this as: Facet 2 (gender) is the facet whose elements are to be identified; the element identifiers for Facet 2 are in the element labels for Facet 1 (examinees); the element identifier for Facet 2 starts in Column 4; the element identifier is 1 column wide. The "Dvalue=" statement, or statements (in case of element identifiers for more than one facet), may be suitably inserted right after the label definition section of the specification file.

Running the MFRM analysis based on the definition of examinee gender as a dummy facet would yield the same Rater-by-Gender Group bias diagram as depicted in Figure 8.4.

8.5 Summary of model variants

As mentioned at the beginning of this chapter, the MFRM approach does not simply refer to a single psychometric model designed for some particular purpose. Rather, MFRM is best understood as a general-purpose measurement approach that comprises a family of models each of which tailored to meet the requirements of a particular assessment context. Only a few instantiations of the general approach have been discussed in the preceding chapters. These and some other commonly used models are outlined in a summary fashion in Table 8.7. The main features of Models A through H, and their interrelations, can briefly be described as follows.

Model A is a kind of baseline model in that it incorporates only two facets: examinees and raters. It is implied that raters use a single scale to evaluate examinee performance. This model is equivalent to a rating scale model as shown in Equation 2.7, but now raters have taken the place of items, and rater severity the place of item difficulty. In most instances, Model A will be an oversimplification, since it takes insufficient account of the facets that usually have an impact in the assessment situation.

Model B is the three-facet rating scale model given in Equation 2.11 and dealt with extensively in the empirical demonstration of the MFRM approach. This model is included in the table for ease of reference.

Model C represents a different assessment context where raters use a single, holistic rating scale to score examinee performance on a number of different tasks (for a comparison of holistic and analytic ratings using a MFRM modeling approach, see Chi, 2001; see also Knoch, 2009a).

The partial credit version of Model B is shown in the equation for Model D, with the partial credit component relating to the scoring criteria (for more detail, see Equation 8.1). That is, the rating scale structure is allowed to vary across criteria.

Table 8.7: Examples of MFRM Models for Rater-Mediated Assessments.

ID	Model Equation	Measurement Objectives
A	$\ln\left[\frac{p_{njk}}{p_{njk-1}}\right]=\theta_n-\alpha_j-\tau_k$	Examinee proficiency (θ_n), rater severity (α_j); constant rating scale structure.
B	$\ln\left[\frac{p_{nijk}}{p_{nijk-1}}\right]=\theta_n-\beta_i-\alpha_j-\tau_k$	Examinee proficiency (θ_n), criterion difficulty (β_i), rater severity (α_j); constant rating scale structure. Detailed discussion in text (see Eq. 2.11).
C	$\ln\left[\frac{p_{nljk}}{p_{nljk-1}}\right]=\theta_n-\delta_l-\alpha_j-\tau_k$	Examinee proficiency (θ_n), task difficulty (δ_l), rater severity (α_j); constant rating scale structure.
D	$\ln\left[\frac{p_{nijk}}{p_{nijk-1}}\right]=\theta_n-\beta_i-\alpha_j-\tau_{ik}$	Examinee proficiency (θ_n), criterion difficulty (β_i), rater severity (α_j); variable structure of the rating scale for criteria. Detailed discussion in text (see Eq. 8.1).
E	$\ln\left[\frac{p_{niljk}}{p_{niljk-1}}\right]=\theta_n-\beta_i-\delta_l-\alpha_J-\tau_{ijk}$	Examinee proficiency (θ_n), criterion difficulty (β_i), task difficulty (δ_l), rater severity (α_j); variable structure of the rating scale for criteria and raters.
F	$\ln\left[\frac{p_{nilvjk}}{p_{nilvjk-1}}\right]=\theta_n-\beta_i-\delta_l-\eta_v-\alpha_j-\tau_k$	Examinee proficiency (θ_n), criterion difficulty (β_i), interviewer difficulty (η_v), task difficulty (δ_l), rater severity (α_j); constant rating scale structure.
G	$\ln\left[\frac{p_{nijk}}{p_{nijk-1}}\right]=\theta_n-\beta_i-\alpha_j-\varphi_{nj}-\tau_k$	Examinee proficiency (θ_n), criterion difficulty (β_i), rater severity (α_j); effect of the interaction between examinees and raters (ϕ_{nj}); constant rating scale structure. Detailed discussion in text (see Eq. 8.4).

ID	Model Equation	Measurement Objectives
H	$\ln\left[\frac{p_{nijk}}{p_{nijk-1}}\right]=\theta_n-\beta_i-\alpha_j-\gamma_g-\varphi_{jg}-\tau_k$	Examinee proficiency (θ_n), criterion difficulty (β_i), rater severity (α_j); effect of examinee gender (subgroup γ_g); effect of rater-by-examinee gender interaction (ϕ_{jg}); constant rating scale structure. Detailed discussion in text (see Eq. 8.6).

Model E combines Models C and D in that criteria and tasks are included in the same equation. Moreover, this model incorporates a partial credit component that refers to both criteria and raters (but not to tasks).

Model F is typical of an investigation on examinee speaking proficiency where live interviewers present several speaking tasks, and raters score examinee performance according to a set of analytic criteria (see also the third introductory example quoted in Chapter 1).

Model G exemplifies the specification of an interaction between examinees and raters, thus forming the basis of an exploratory interaction analysis (for more detail, see Equation 8.4).

The final model in the summary table, Model H, illustrates a confirmatory interaction analysis. The model includes an examinee background variable (i.e., gender) and allows the researcher to study an interaction between examinee gender and raters (for more detail, see Equation 8.6).

Regarding the models that are suited for studying possible rater bias, a word of caution appears appropriate (C. M. Myford, personal communication, February 24, 2015). When conducting a bias analysis using demographic variables of examinees, it is sometimes advisable to view the results of such an analysis as tentative and needing further scrutiny. For example, if a researcher were running a bias analysis and found that a rater did not exercise a uniform level of severity when rating examinees from different demographic groups (e.g., gender, age, or ethnic groups), the researcher might want to be careful before concluding that a particular rater showed evidence of bias. It could well be that the results were due to the fact that the rater had only rated a small number of examinees in one or more subgroups. In cases like this more data on larger samples of examinee subgroups need to be gathered and subjected to a bias analysis.

9. Special Issues

The MFRM approach to rater-mediated assessment raises a number of more specialized issues, some of which concern the design of collecting many-facet data; others relate to benefits that accrue from conducting a MFRM analysis in terms of facilitating detailed rater feedback or informing standard setting. This chapter deals with design issues first, since they figure prominently in any kind of many-facet data analysis. Then, some of the practical benefits a MFRM approach holds for providing feedback to raters and for evaluating judgments gathered in the context of standard-setting studies are discussed. A more technical section highlights key differences between the MFRM approach and CTT-based generalizability theory (G-theory). The chapter concludes with a brief description of computer software suited to implement MFRM models or various kinds of model extensions.

9.1 Rating designs

In rater-mediated assessment, great care needs to be taken concerning the design according to which the rating data are collected. For example, when raters provide scores for the performances of examinees on a number of tasks, questions like these may arise: Should all raters score all examinees, or would it be sufficient if subsets of raters each scored a particular subset of examinees? What is a reasonable number of raters per examinee, how many examinees should each rater score, and should each rater score examinee performance on each task? With only a few raters scoring a subset of examinees, how should raters be assigned to examinees in order to make sure that all elements of the facets involved, that is, raters, examinees, and tasks, can be represented in the same frame of reference?

To begin with, MFRM modeling is generally robust against mistakes in the implementation of a rating design. In particular, those in charge of the assessment program may initiate the MFRM analysis as soon as data collection begins (see Linacre & Wright, 2002). This way, mistakes in the implementation of the rating design, or problematic behavior of raters, can be identified and corrected before the rating process is completed. If necessary, a conspicuous rater can be defined as "two raters", one providing ratings before remediation and the other after remediation (J. M. Linacre, personal communication, March 27, 2009).

Generally, the choice of a particular rating design depends on a mix of measurement and practical considerations (Du & Brown, 2000; Engelhard, 1997; Hombo, Donoghue, & Thayer, 2001; Myford & Wolfe, 2000; Sykes, Ito, & Wang, 2008). First, other things being equal, the more data are collected, the higher the measurement precision of model parameters will be. For example, the larger the number of raters is per examinee, the more precise are the estimates of examinee proficiency and task difficulty.

Second, even large subsets of raters per examinee do not guard against running into serious measurement problems when the rating design does not provide for sufficient links between facet elements. This crucial design aspect concerns the *connectedness* of the resulting data set. A connected data set is one in which a network of links exists through which every element that is involved in producing an observation is directly or indirectly connected to every other element of the same assessment context (Engelhard, 1997; Linacre & Wright, 2002; Wright & Stone, 1979). Lack of connectedness among elements of a particular facet (e.g., among raters) would make it impossible to calibrate all elements of that facet on the same scale; that is, the measures constructed for these elements (e.g., rater severity measures) could not be directly compared. Ways to remedy an observed lack of connectedness are discussed later.

Third, in many assessment situations, particularly in large-scale assessments, practical considerations heavily narrow the choice of a rating design. Such considerations typically refer to time constraints, reasonable rater workload, and budget issues.

Table 9.1 illustrates the basic structure of rating designs that are suited to highlight some of the measurement and practical considerations just mentioned. Each of these designs refers to a hypothetical assessment situation involving 10 examinees, 4 raters, and 2 tasks. Needless to say, operational rating sessions for calibrating examinees, raters, and tasks would comprise much larger sets of examinees and, possibly, raters and/or tasks, as well (see, for a detailed discussion of data collection designs in measurement contexts involving two facets, Kolen, 2007; Kolen & Brennan, 2004; Wolfe, 2000).

Table 9.1: Illustration of Rating Designs for Three-Facet Rater-Mediated Performance Assessments.

		Examinee									
Rater	**Task**	**1**	**2**	**3**	**4**	**5**	**6**	**7**	**8**	**9**	**10**
A. Complete (Fully Crossed) Design											
1	1, 2	✓	✓	✓	✓	✓	✓	✓	✓	✓	✓
2	1, 2	✓	✓	✓	✓	✓	✓	✓	✓	✓	✓
3	1, 2	✓	✓	✓	✓	✓	✓	✓	✓	✓	✓
4	1, 2	✓	✓	✓	✓	✓	✓	✓	✓	✓	✓

Rater	Task	Examinee									
		1	2	3	4	5	6	7	8	9	10
B. Incomplete Design – Connected											
1	1, 2	✓	✓		✓	✓	✓		✓	✓	✓
2	1, 2	✓	✓	✓		✓	✓	✓		✓	✓
3	1, 2		✓	✓	✓		✓	✓	✓		✓
4	1, 2	✓		✓	✓	✓		✓	✓	✓	
C. Incomplete Design – Connected											
1	1, 2	✓			✓			✓			✓
2	1, 2					✓			✓		✓
3	1, 2			✓			✓				✓
4	1, 2		✓							✓	✓
D. Incomplete Design – Disconnected											
1	1, 2	✓	✓	✓	✓	✓	✓				
2	1, 2	✓	✓	✓	✓	✓	✓				
3	1, 2							✓	✓	✓	✓
4	1, 2							✓	✓	✓	✓
E. Incomplete, spiral design – Connected											
1	1	✓	✓	✓	✓	✓	✓	✓	✓	✓	✓
2	2	✓	✓	✓	✓	✓	✓	✓	✓	✓	✓
3	1	✓	✓	✓	✓	✓	✓	✓	✓	✓	✓
4	2	✓	✓	✓	✓	✓	✓	✓	✓	✓	✓

Note. Designs A through E refer to a simplified assessment situation where 10 examinees respond to 2 tasks each and 4 raters provide scores on a single, holistic rating scale. Each ✓ designates an observation.

The first design, Rating Design A, according to which all raters score all examinees on all tasks, is an example of a *complete* or *fully crossed* design. Each tick mark (✓) in the design notation refers to an observation, response, or score available for parameter estimation. A complete design is the optimum design from a measurement point of view since it leads to the highest precision of model parameter estimates possible and to a data set that has not a single missing link. Yet, conceivably, this design is rarely, if ever, practical in real assessment situations.

More practical is Rating Design B. This is an example of an *incomplete* design, which simultaneously satisfies the measurement constraint of yielding a connected data set. Therefore, Design B is also called a *connected* (or *linked*) design: Each rater scores only a subset of examinees, and each examinee is scored by only three out of the four raters, yet all elements of all three facets are linked to each other in a common network. For example, Rater 1 is linked to Rater 3 through common ratings of Examinees 2, 4, 6, 8, and 10. Conversely, each examinee is linked to each other examinee (e.g., Examinee 1 to Examinee 2, or Examinee 3 to Examinee 10) through ratings by at least two common raters.

A further reduction in each rater's workload is achieved through incomplete Rating Design C. Each rater has to score only three or four examinees. Moreover, each examinee, except for Examinee 10, is scored by exactly one rater. Compared to complete Design A, the number of observations in Design C is reduced by 34%. Yet, since Examinee 10 is scored by all four raters, the connectedness condition is preserved.

In contrast to Designs A through C, use of Rating Design D would result in a data set with insufficient links. This is referred to as a *disconnected* design. Though more observations are available than in Design C, the specific way of assigning raters to examinees that follows from Design D generates two *disjoint* or *disconnected subsets* of raters: Subset 1 contains Raters 1 and 2, and Subset 2 contains Raters 3 and 4. In a case like this, only measures in the same subset are directly comparable; that is, it would be misleading to compare the severity measures for Raters 1 and 3, or those for Raters 2 and 4. For example, when Rater 1 turned out to award, on average, lower scores than Rater 3, it would remain unclear whether this was due to higher severity of Rater 1 or to lower average proficiency of the examinees rated by Rater 1, as compared to examinees rated by Rater 3. Put differently, rater severity and examinee proficiency would be confounded.

The last design shown in Table 9.1 is a special variant of an incomplete, connected design that reduces the rater workload by assigning raters to score examinee performance on a subset of tasks only. Rating Design E exemplifies a *spiral* design (Hombo et al., 2001). Since performance on each task is scored by a different set of raters (Task 1 is scored by Raters 1 and 3, Task 2 is scored by Raters 2 and 4), this design is also called a *nested* design; that is, raters are nested within tasks.

As an instructive example of a real rating design consider again the sample data from the writing performance assessment described in Section 2.2.2. One of the 18 raters (Rater 06) was deliberately chosen to rate two essays each randomly drawn from the subsets of essays already rated by each of the other 17 raters.

These third ratings yielded a rating design similar in structure to Design C (Table 9.1); that is, a design that is incomplete yet connected. The connecting element in Design C is Examinee 10. In the operational rating design on which the sample data analysis was based, Rater 06 provided the required connection. To illustrate, dropping this rater from the rater panel would lead to a disconnected design, with the group of raters split into three disjoint subsets as follows: Raters 01, 03, 08, 12, 13, 14, and 16 formed Subset 1; Raters 05, 07, 09, 10, 11, 15, 17, and 18 formed Subset 2; and Raters 02 and 04 formed Subset 3. Refer to Table 3.1 to see that raters in the same subset are linked to each other, but raters from different subsets are not. For example, there is no link between Rater 01 (Subset 1) and Rater 05 (Subset 2), whereas Rater 01 (Subset 1) is directly linked to Rater 14, and indirectly linked to Rater 03 (same subset) via Raters 14, 08, and 12; that is, the indirect link between Raters 01 and 03 is established by rater pairs 14/08, 08/12, and, finally, 12/03.

As this example suggests, one way to remedy an apparent lack of connectedness that manifested itself during the process of data collection (and concomitant data analysis) would be to ask one rater, or a small number of raters, to rate samples of performances that were placed into disconnected subsets. Raters coming from the group of operational raters would thus have to provide ratings in addition to their normal workload; raters from outside the group would need to provide ratings of a sufficiently large number of carefully chosen performances in order not to create disconnectedness again. Alternatively, if the lack of connectedness was due to examinees responding to two or more independent sets of items or tasks, a small number of examinees could be asked to respond also to a sample of items (or tasks) that were common to these sets.

Alternatively, when lack of connectedness was diagnosed only *after* having completed the rating process, a procedure called *group anchoring* (Linacre, 2014b) may help resolving the problem. For example, when the occurrence of disconnected subsets was due to administering different sets of items to independent groups of examinees, and the sets of items were deliberately constructed to be of the same overall difficulty, then these sets could reasonably be anchored at the same average difficulty measure (usually 0 logits). Similarly, when independent groups of raters provided ratings of a large sample of performances, and these performances were allocated to each individual rater at random (i.e., irrespective of group membership), thus yielding rater groups that were randomly equivalent, the different groups of raters could be equated by assigning the same average severity measure to each rater across groups.

There are at least two more group-anchoring strategies that may be used depending on circumstances (C. M. Myford, personal communication, January 22, 2011). The first one is to set the mean severity of two (or more) disconnected subgroups of raters at 0 logits. That way each rater's level of severity within each subgroup is allowed to float, relative to that set mean (i.e., you are not assigning the same severity measure to each rater). With this strategy, the assumption is that the subgroups of raters have the same mean severity, but not that they each exercised the same level of severity. A related strategy is to anchor the mean proficiency of two (or more) disconnected subgroups of examinees at 0 logits. Using this strategy, each examinee's level of proficiency within each subgroup is allowed to float, relative to that set mean. The assumption here is that the subgroups of examinees have the same mean proficiency, but not that they all were equally proficient.

Note also that FACETS automatically tests for connectedness in the data being analyzed. In case disconnected subsets are found the program produces a corresponding message and reports subsets of connected elements. The user may then request a subset group-anchor file in which FACETS will suggest appropriate group-anchoring strategies that could solve the disconnected subsets problem, providing directions about how to implement each strategy.

9.2 Rater feedback

A MFRM analysis does not only provide the basis for reporting assessment results to examinees that are corrected for differences in rater severity, but also has an important role to play in rater training and rater monitoring activities. As mentioned before, rater training can be quite effective in terms of increasing within-rater consistency. Rater monitoring helps to evaluate the functioning of the raters as a group, and to identify individual rating patterns that are conspicuous in some way or another.

An increase in within-rater consistency may be achieved through various forms of *individualized* feedback (but see Knoch, 2011). Each rater would be given detailed information on his or her rating behavior, distracting attention away from stressful and mostly futile comparisons with other raters in the group. Results of a MFRM analysis provide a suitable basis for compiling this kind of feedback (e.g., Hoskens & Wilson, 2001; Knoch et al., 2007; O'Sullivan & Rignall, 2007; Stahl & Lunz, 1996; Wigglesworth, 1993). Stahl and Lunz (1996) put it this way:

> Emphasis on intra- rather than inter-judge consistency removes a great deal of stress from the judging situation. Judges need not worry about whether they are too "hard" or

> too "easy", whether they are grading the same way as their peers or not. Rather, judges focus on applying their expertise as honestly as possible. (p. 123)

Individualized feedback that is communicated to raters may consist of one or more of the following components: (a) a particular rater's severity or leniency measure (suitably transformed to a familiar scale; see below), (b) a severity map showing the distribution of severity measures, or fair rater averages, within the respective group of raters (particularly useful are bar graphs, where each targeted rater is clearly identified and represented by a different bar; see Figure 9.1), (c) the degree of within-rater consistency as measured by rater infit and/or outfit indices, (d) frequency of usage of rating scale categories, and (e) quality control charts (or bias diagrams) portraying the deviations of the rater's ratings from model expectations with respect to examinees, criteria, tasks, items, or whatever other facets are considered important in the feedback process.

The rationale behind individualized feedback is that raters are construed as experts who bring individual standards and expectations to the assessment context, yet at the same time are willing to learn more about their rating patterns. Each rater is allowed his or her own level of severity, as long as this level is applied in a self-consistent manner, faithfully reflecting the underlying construct. To this end, each piece of information conveyed to raters should come in a form that is sufficiently differentiated, easy to grasp, and supportive of each rater's efforts at becoming, or staying, a consistent rater. That is, rater feedback should be encouraging and motivating, providing information where to take corrective action when necessary.

Rasch severity measures that are reported in logits contain decimals and negatives and can range from $-\infty$ to $+\infty$. In particular, severity measures reported in logits will be negative for one half of the rater group and positive for the other half (when, as usual, the rater facet is centered, i.e., the mean severity measure is constrained to be zero). These properties of the logit scale may be confusing to those unfamiliar with measurement results being reported in the standard unit of measurement (i.e., logits).

Fig. 9.1: Bar graph providing feedback to Rater 05. The graph shows the distribution of rater severities in the group of raters expressed as fair averages (shown along the vertical axis). Raters are ordered from left to right by increasing leniency.

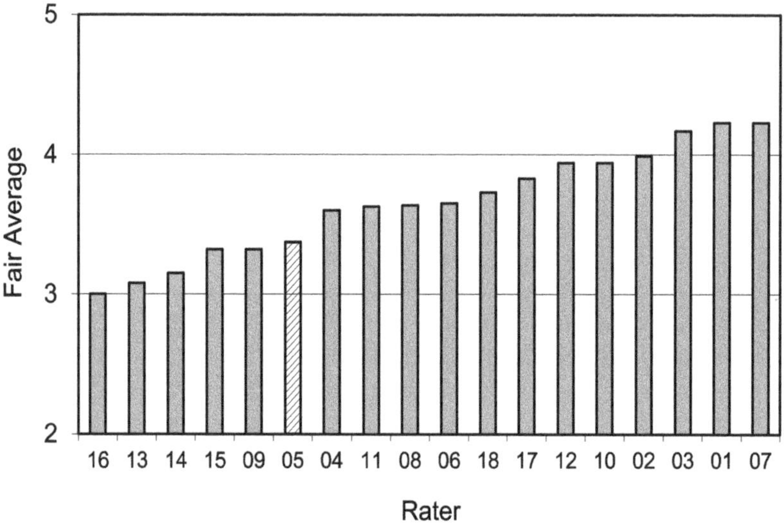

Therefore, when conveying severity information to raters, results may rather be reported using some sort of qualitatively ordered category system (e.g., *highly lenient, lenient, average, severe, highly severe*). Consistency information could be coded in an analogous fashion (e.g., from *highly consistent* to *highly inconsistent*).

More detailed and informative feedback to raters would make use of fair averages. As discussed earlier, fair averages highlight differences between raters in direct reference to the rating scale, or scales, used during the assessment; that is, fair rater averages show rater severity measures in the raw-score metric. Figure 9.1 illustrates one way of providing this kind of feedback to Rater 05.

Another way is to linearly transform the logit scale. For example, if a scale of severity measures with the familiar range of 0 to 100 is desired, with the lowest measure equal to 0 and the highest measure equal to 100, then the following transformation of logits taken from the rater measurement results would yield the new scale (e.g., Smith, 2004; Wright & Stone, 1979):

$$\hat{\alpha}_j^* = m + s \cdot \hat{\alpha}_j, \tag{9.1}$$

where

$$m = 0 - (s \cdot \min_j), \tag{9.2}$$

and

$$s = 100 / (\max_j - \min_j). \tag{9.3}$$

In Equation 9.1, $\hat{\alpha}_j^*$ is the severity estimate for rater j on the new scale, m is the location factor for determining the new scale origin, s is the spacing factor for determining the new scale unit, and $\hat{\alpha}_j$ is the severity estimate for rater j on the old scale (i.e., the logit scale); $\min_j$ and $\max_j$ refer to the smallest and largest severity estimate (in logits), respectively.

Finally, based on the spacing factor s, the standard error for the rescaled rater severity estimate, that is, SE_j^*, is computed as follows:

$$SE_j^* = s \cdot SE_j. \tag{9.4}$$

Referring to the rater measurement results reported in Table 5.1, and using Equations 9.1 to 9.3, the severity measure for Rater 13 (2.09 logits, SE = 0.20) becomes 93.31 points on the new scale (i.e., m = 48.27, s = 21.55); rounding down yields a severity measure of 93 points on the 0–100 scale. A value such as this one is generally much easier to communicate than the original logit value. Using Equation 9.4, the standard error of the rescaled severity measure for Rater 13 becomes 4.31.[14]

9.3 Standard setting

Standard setting refers to the process of establishing one or more cut scores on a test (Cizek, 2006; Cizek & Bunch, 2007; Hambleton & Pitoniak, 2006; Kaftandjieva, 2004, 2010). Cut scores are used to divide a distribution of test scores into two or more categories of performance, representing distinct levels of knowledge, competence, or proficiency in a given domain. Thus, examinees may be categorized as *pass* or *fail*, or may be placed into a greater number of ordered performance categories, with labels such as *basic*, *proficient*, and *advanced*. When

14 In an analogous fashion, examinee proficiency measures, item difficulty measures, etc., expressed in logits, can be linearly transformed to yield more familiar scales, such as the 0–100 scale. Transformations of this kind can be performed in FACETS using the "Umean=" command (in the rater severity rescaling example: "Umean=48.27,21.55").

setting cut scores on language tests, the categories are typically taken from the CEFR six-level global scale (Council of Europe, 2001), ranging from *basic user* (subdivided into levels A1, A2) through *intermediate user* (B1, B2) to *proficient user* (C1, C2).

According to Hambleton and Pitoniak (2006), standard setting is a "blend of judgment, psychometrics, and practicality" (p. 435). The authors characterized judgments provided by panelists as the "cornerstone" on which the resulting cut scores are based (in the context of standard setting raters are often called *panelists, judges*, or *subject matter experts*). Due to the high stakes involved in many decisions that derive from the application of cut scores, it is imperative to evaluate the standard-setting process and the appropriateness of the final outcomes. The *Standards for Educational and Psychological Testing* (American Educational Research Association, American Psychological Association, & National Council on Measurement in Education, 2014) discussed sources of validity evidence required to argue for proposed score interpretations that involve one or more cut scores (i.e., Standards 5.21–5.23).

One particularly important source of validity evidence refers to the consistency within and between judges. For example, judges have been shown to employ different standards when judging the difficulty of items or placing examinees into performance categories (e.g., Longford, 1996; Van Nijlen & Janssen, 2008). These interjudge differences need to be taken into account before determining cut scores. MFRM models are well-suited to do this. Moreover, MFRM models can be used to provide estimates of cut scores in a variety of testing and assessment contexts. In the following, I briefly elaborate on MFRM applications to two frequently used standard-setting procedures, the *Angoff method* or, more precisely, the "unmodified" Angoff approach (Cizek & Bunch, 2007; Plake & Cizek, 2012), and the *bookmark method* (Lewis, Mitzel, Mercado, & Schulz, 2012; Mitzel, Lewis, Patz, & Green, 2001).

In the Angoff method (Angoff, 1971), judges are presented with a number of dichotomous items and asked the following question for each item: Out of 100 minimally competent examinees, how many would answer this item correctly? Viewed from a measurement perspective, the ratings obtained can be modeled as outcomes of binomial trials; that is, the number of independent trials (m) is fixed at "100", and the judges are asked to count the number of "successes", which corresponds to the number of minimally competent examinees who would answer the item correctly. The following MFRM model can be used to analyze these data (Engelhard & Anderson, 1998; Engelhard & Cramer, 1997):

$$\ln\left[\frac{p_{jix}}{p_{jix-1}}\right] = \alpha_j - \beta_i - \tau_x, \qquad (9.5)$$

where

p_{jix}	=	probability of judge *j* giving a count of *x* on item *i*,
p_{jix-1}	=	probability of judge *j* giving a count of *x* – 1 on item *i*,
α_j	=	judged minimal competence (severity) for judge *j*,
β_i	=	judged difficulty for item *i*,
τ_x	=	judged difficulty of giving a count of *x* relative to *x* – 1.

Parameter α_j in Equation 9.5 is different in meaning from the rater severity parameter discussed earlier. This parameter now represents the severity of a particular judge's view of minimal competence required to answer item *i* correctly; that is, a severe judge would give a small count of minimally competent examinees answering that item correctly, whereas a lenient judge would give a large count. Furthermore, β_i in Equation 9.5 refers to the *judged* difficulty of item *i*; that is, a difficult item would be given small counts by the judges, as compared to an easy item.[15]

Based on the model given in Equation 9.5, statistical indicators described in previous chapters of this book, such as separation, fit, and bias statistics, can be used to analyze the psychometric quality of the judges' ratings. The Wright map would provide a particularly instructive portrayal of the measurement results for the standard-setting judges and the items. As to the judge facet, the map would show the location of the minimally competent examinee as viewed by the judges, where a higher location represents a higher minimal competence required to answer items correctly (i.e., corresponding to a severe judge's view of minimal competence). With regard to the item facet, the map would show the location of each item in terms of its judged difficulty, where a higher location represents a lower count of examinees answering the item correctly.

In addition, studying the relation between judged item difficulties and empirical item difficulties (e.g., item difficulties derived from operational test administrations) may yield valuable evidence regarding the validity of the

15 The binomial trials model reduces to the Rasch model for dichotomous data if $m = 1$; that is, $x = 0$ or 1 (Wright & Masters, 1982).

standard-setting procedure (Baghaei, 2007; Kaliski et al., 2013; Taube, 1997; Verheggen, Muijtjens, van Os, & Schuwirth, 2008).

A different kind of MFRM model is called for when evaluating a standard setting where panelists provide judgments on the *level of performance* needed to succeed on each of a number of items. The test or assessment may contain a mixture of selected-response (e.g., multiple-choice) and constructed-response items, and the judges may be asked to consider a single level or multiple levels of performance.

For example, consider a test containing 60 multiple-choice items designed to assess four performance levels. In the bookmark method (Mitzel et al., 2001), judges would be presented with a booklet consisting of the set of 60 items, one item per page, with items ordered from easy to hard. Judges would be asked, for each level of performance, to place a bookmark on the first page in the booklet at which they believe the probability of answering the item correctly drops below a 2/3 chance (i.e., below a .67 probability). Thus, panelists would have to place three bookmarks in their booklet, each one identifying a cut-off between two adjacent performance levels. Judges are usually asked to repeat this marking procedure two times, each marking session constituting a separate round (see, for a detailed description of the bookmark method, Lewis et al., 2012).

Each bookmark placement sorts the set of items into one of four performance categories. Bookmark placements can thus be construed as judgments or ratings of items on a four-category performance scale. A MFRM model suited to the analysis of such bookmark ratings could be defined as follows (Engelhard, 2007b, 2008b, 2011):

$$\ln\left[\frac{p_{jirk}}{p_{jirk-1}}\right] = \alpha_j - \beta_i - \rho_r - \tau_{rk}, \qquad (9.6)$$

where

p_{jirk}	=	probability of judge *j* giving a bookmark rating of *k* on item *i* for round *r*,
p_{jirk-1}	=	probability of judge *j* giving a bookmark rating of *k* – 1 on item *i* for round *r*,
α_j	=	judged performance level (severity) for judge *j*,
β_i	=	judged difficulty of item *i*,
ρ_r	=	judged performance level for round *r*,
τ_{rk}	=	judged performance standard in round *r* for bookmark rating of *k* relative to *k* – 1.

The model given in Equation 9.6 is an example of a three-facet partial credit model, where the partial-credit component applies to the *round facet*; that is, this model allows the judged performance standards, or cut scores, to vary by round. Specifically, inclusion of the round facet makes it possible to study changes in between-rater differences in judged performance level as well as changes in within-rater judgment consistency from one round to the next. The final Rasch-based cut scores may be defined as the category coefficients, τ_{rk}, estimated for the last round (possibly after removal of misfitting judges). In order to provide evidence concerning the validity of the measurement approach, the Rasch-based cut scores, after appropriate rescaling, may be compared to the observed cut scores determined by the usual bookmark procedure (e.g., Engelhard, 2011).

There is a broad range of MFRM applications to Angoff, bookmark, and other standard-setting procedures (e.g., Engelhard & Gordon, 2000; Engelhard & Stone, 1998; Hsieh, 2013; Kaliski et al., 2013; Kecker & Eckes, 2010; Kozaki, 2004, 2010; Lumley, Lynch, & McNamara, 1994; Lunz, 2000; Stone, 2006; Stone, Beltyukova, & Fox, 2008). In each of these studies, the MFRM modeling approach proved valuable for the purposes of evaluating standard-setting data and/or setting cut scores on various kinds of tests and assessments.

On a more cautionary note, an important aim of many standard-setting procedures is to reach consensus among judges before deciding on the cut scores. Yet, as discussed earlier, implicitly or explicitly forcing judges into agreement is bound to create some degree of dependence among judges that may pose problems for interpreting results from a MFRM analysis. The Rasch measurement approach basically construes raters or judges as independent experts, with each judgment providing a new piece of information about the location of an item (or an examinee) on the latent continuum (see Section 5.3). It may thus be reasonable not to perform MFRM analyses in the later stages of standard setting where judges can be assumed to gravitate toward the group mean.

9.4 Generalizability theory (G-theory)

Chapter 3 introduced the conceptual–psychometric framework underlying the MFRM approach. This framework distinguished between proximal facets having an immediate impact on assessment scores, and distal facets the influence of which may be more indirect. Much the same facets are considered in the psychometric approach of generalizability theory (G-theory), albeit in a fundamentally different way. G-theory allows investigators to study the relative effects of each of these facets and their manifold interactions in an effort to examine the dependability of behavioral measures, in particular test scores or assessment outcomes.

In this section, I first present basic concepts and elements of G-theory and then discuss points of divergence from the MFRM approach.

Fig. 9.2: Decomposition of observed score variance within G-theory.

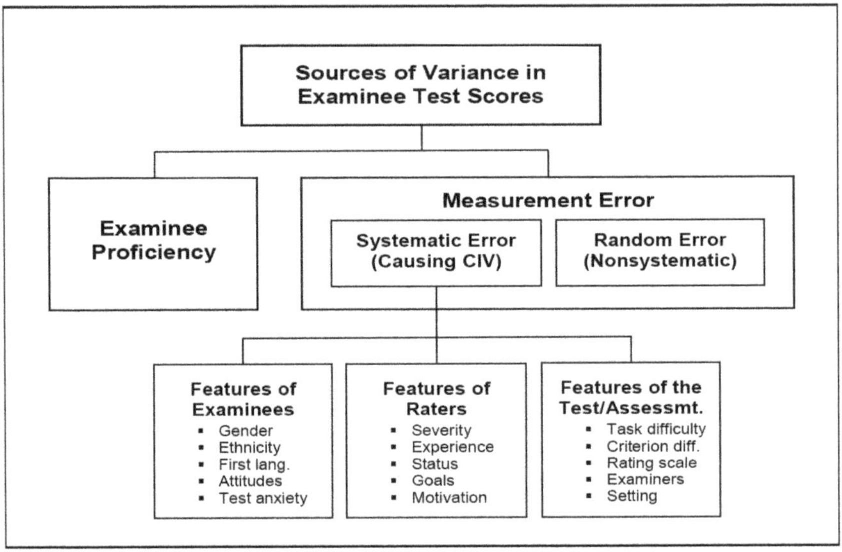

G-theory (Brennan, 2001; Cronbach, Gleser, Nanda, & Rajaratnam, 1972) has its roots in classical test theory (CTT). In CTT, all measurement error is assumed to be random. Expressed in terms of variances, CTT partitions the variance in observed scores into two parts: (a) the variance that is thought to be systematic (i.e., true variance), and (b) the variance that is thought to be random (i.e., error variance). Whereas true variance is caused by differences between examinees in the proficiency being measured, error variance is caused by anything else that makes an examinee's observed score differ from his or her true score.

In contrast, G-theory rejects the notion of a single undifferentiated measurement error and rather posits that measurement error arises from *multiple* sources (Brennan, 2011). Specifically, G-theory aims at estimating the magnitude of each source separately and provides a strategy for optimizing the reliability of behavioral measurements. One source of measurement error is random error; other sources refer to facets contributing to construct-irrelevant variance, such as features of examinees other than the proficiency being measured, features of raters, and features of the test or assessment procedure. In addition, G-theory allows to address interactions between examinee proficiency and sources of systematic measurement error.

Figure 9.2 portrays the decomposition of the observed variance in examinee test or assessment scores into true variance and error variance, which is further decomposed into variance due to systematic error (i.e., construct-irrelevant variance, or CIV, for short) and variance due to random error. Also shown are three typical classes of potential sources of systematic measurement error, each explained using examples that represent a mix of distal and proximal facets discussed earlier (for an overview of systematic errors associated with CIV, see Haladyna & Downing, 2004). Note that in the G-theory framework, potential sources of systematic measurement error are called *facets*, the levels of these facets are called *conditions*, and the source of variance that is of interest (normally examinee proficiency) is called the *object of measurement*.

In G-theory, an observed score is conceived of as a sample from a *universe of admissible observations*. This universe is defined in terms of the facets that an investigator decides to be of relevance to the assessment context. For example, any experienced and well-trained rater may be considered an admissible condition of measurement for the rater facet. Similarly, any criterion designed to capture a distinct feature of examinee performance may be considered an admissible condition of measurement for the criterion facet. In addition, any one of the possible combinations of raters and criteria may be accepted as meaningful. In this instance, the universe of admissible observations would be described as being *fully crossed*; that is, all examinees' responses to a given task would be rated by the same raters on the same set of criteria.

A G-theory analysis proceeds in two stages. In the first stage, called a *generalizability study* (G-study), estimates of *variance components* associated with a universe of admissible observations are obtained. The relative magnitudes of the estimated variance components provide information about the different sources of measurement error.

In the second stage, called a *decision study* (D-study), variance component information from a G-study is used to design a measurement procedure that minimizes error for a particular purpose. Technically speaking, a D-study specifies a *universe of generalization*, which is the universe to which an investigator, or a decision-maker, wants to generalize based on the information obtained in a G-study (for detailed discussions of G-study and D-study designs, see Brennan, 2001, 2011; Marcoulides, 2000; Shavelson & Webb, 1991).

To illustrate the G-theory approach, consider the sample data once again: There was a high percentage of missing observations (i.e., 1,944 actual observations out of 16,578 possible observations, or 88.3% missing data) and the sample size varied for each element (level) of the rater facet; that is, each rater rated a different number of essays. Thus, the design of the writing assessment study was *unbalanced* in a way that made the data unwieldy for a standard G-theory analysis (Chiu, 2001; Chiu & Wolfe, 2002). Just to get a glimpse of the rationale and procedure of G-theory, though, I restricted the following example to a small portion of the data where two raters, discussed in detail previously (i.e., Rater 13 and Rater 03), rated each of 21 essays on the three criteria, making the data design a fully crossed (i.e., balanced) one. These data were analyzed by means of the computer program GENOVA (Version 3.1; Crick & Brennan, 2001).

In the present G-study, the observed score x_{nij} awarded to examinee n on criterion i by rater j can be expressed in terms of the following linear model:

$$x_{nij} = \mu + \nu_n + \nu_i + \nu_j + \nu_{ni} + \nu_{nj} + \nu_{ij} + \nu_{nij,e}, \tag{9.7}$$

where μ is the grand mean in the population (of examinees) and universe (of criteria crossed with raters) and ν denotes any one of the effects for this design: main effects attributable to examinee n (ν_n), criterion i (ν_i), and rater j (ν_j), as well as interaction effects between examinee n and criterion i (ν_{ni}), between examinee n and rater j (ν_{nj}), and between criterion i and rater j (ν_{ij}); $\nu_{nij,e}$ denotes the residual effect.[16] For example, the main effect attributable to examinee n can be expressed as:

$$\nu_n = \mu_n - \mu, \tag{9.8}$$

where μ_n is the *universe score* for examinee n. The universe score is an examinee's average (expected) score over the entire universe of admissible observations.

The total variance of the observed scores given by Equation 9.7 can be decomposed into seven independent variance components:

$$\sigma^2_{x_{nij}} = \sigma^2_n + \sigma^2_i + \sigma^2_j + \sigma^2_{ni} + \sigma^2_{nj} + \sigma^2_{ij} + \sigma^2_{nij,e}. \tag{9.9}$$

Results of the G-study comprise estimates of the variance components shown in Equation 9.9. Note that these components are associated with single observations (e.g., the relative effect of a single criterion or a single rater on an examinee's score), as opposed to average scores over criteria and/or raters, which are

16 Since there is only one observation for each combination of examinee, criterion, and rater, it is impossible to estimate the three-way interaction component and the error component separately (i.e., the three-way interaction and error components are confounded); hence, they are lumped together and referred to as the residual effect.

addressed in D-studies. Estimates of variance components are obtained by means of analysis of variance (ANOVA) procedures (e.g., Myers et al., 2010). For the sample data considered here, the estimated variance components are shown in Table 9.2; also shown are the results for three D-studies.

The variance component attributed to examinees (0.569) accounts for 40.3% of the total observed score variance, indicating that examinees differed considerably in writing proficiency. All other variance components represent sources of measurement error. The highest of these components refers to the rater facet (0.491) and accounts for 34.8% of the observed variance. This result is in accord with what we already know about Rater 13 and Rater 03 from the MFRM analysis; that is, the rater effect is due to pronounced differences in these raters' severity.

In order to examine whether an increase in the number of raters and/or an increase in the number of criteria would have the desired effect of reducing the proportion of error variance, various D-studies can be specified. For the purposes of illustration, Table 9.2 portrays the results of three such D-studies.

Each D-study provides two types of error variance. The first type is the *relative error variance*, which corresponds to relative decisions; that is, decisions about the rank ordering of examinees (norm-referenced decisions). In this instance, all the sources of variation due to interactions that include examinees are considered measurement error. The second type is the *absolute error variance*, which corresponds to absolute decisions; that is, decisions about the level of performance (criterion-referenced decisions). Here, the error variance includes all the sources of variation, except that due to examinees.

Relative and absolute error variances give rise to two reliability-like coefficients. The first one is the *generalizability coefficient*, which is given by:

$$\rho^2 = \frac{\sigma_n^2}{\sigma_n^2 + \sigma_{\mathrm{rel}}^2}, \tag{9.10}$$

where σ_n^2 is the source of variation due to examinees (i.e., universe-score variance) and σ_{rel}^2 is the relative error variance.

Table 9.2: Results of the G-Study and Alternative D-Studies.

			Alternative D-Studies					
Source of Variation	**G-Study**		**1**		**2**		**3**	
Number of Criteria	1		3		6		3	
Number of Raters	1		2		2		4	
	EVC	%	EVC	%	EVC	%	EVC	%
Examinees ($N = 21$)	0.569	40.3	0.569	60.9	0.569	62.3	0.569	74.5
Criteria ($I = 3$)	0.046	3.3	0.015	1.6	0.008	0.9	0.015	2.0
Raters ($J = 2$)	0.491	34.8	0.245	26.2	0.245	26.8	0.123	16.1
Examinees × Criteria (*ni*)	0.024	1.7	0.008	0.9	0.004	0.4	0.008	1.0
Examinees × Raters (*nj*)	0.152	10.8	0.076	8.1	0.076	8.3	0.038	5.0
Criteria × Raters (*ij*)	0.000	0.0	0.000	0.0	0.000	0.0	0.000	0.0
Residual (*nij,e*)	0.129	9.1	0.021	2.2	0.011	1.2	0.011	1.4
Relative error variance			0.105		0.091		0.057	
Generalizability coefficient (ρ^2)			0.844		0.863		0.909	
Absolute error variance			0.366		0.344		0.195	
Dependability coefficient (Φ)			0.608		0.623		0.745	

Note. EVC = estimated variance component. % = percentage of variance.

The second reliability-like coefficient is the *dependability coefficient*, which is given by:

$$\Phi = \frac{\sigma_n^2}{\sigma_n^2 + \sigma_{\text{abs}}^2}, \qquad (9.11)$$

where σ_n^2 is defined as above and σ_{abs}^2 is the absolute error variance.

As can be seen from the values in the bottom part of Table 9.2, the smallest relative and absolute error variances, and, as a consequence, the highest coefficients of generalizability and dependability, respectively, were obtained in D-study 3. Thus, as compared to D-study 1, doubling the number of raters

(D-study 3) led to a considerably higher reliability of the measurement procedure than doubling the number of criteria (D-study 2).[17]

G-theory has been compared to the MFRM modeling approach in a number of studies conducted in the field of language assessment (e.g., Akiyama, 2001; Bachman, Lynch, & Mason, 1995; Kim & Wilson, 2009; Kozaki, 2004; Lunz & Schumacker, 1997; Lynch & McNamara, 1998; MacMillan, 2000; Sudweeks, Reeve, & Bradshaw, 2005) and elsewhere (e.g., Iramaneerat, Yudkowsky, Myford, & Downing, 2008; Smith & Kulikowich, 2004). Each of these studies looked at the basic measurement implications of both approaches and pinpointed differences in the specific way each approach deals with unwanted variability in rater-mediated assessments. Some of the major differences are summarized below (for a more detailed discussion, see Linacre, 1996a, 2001).

First, the ANOVA procedures used in a G-theory analysis presuppose that the input data have the properties of an interval scale, but actually ratings are more likely to be ordinal. Moreover, G-theory focuses on an examinee's total score as the unit of analysis and expresses this score in the ordinal metric of the original ratings. In contrast, the measures that result from a MFRM analysis (examinee proficiency measures, rater severity measures, etc.) have the properties of a linear, equal-interval scale if the data fit the model. Therefore, these measures are suitable for the calculation of means and variances.

Second, G-theory does not adjust observed scores for differences in rater severity, differences in criterion difficulty, or differences in measures relating to some other facet. G-theory aims to estimate the error variance associated with examinee raw scores in order to provide information on how to improve the reliability of the ratings. As demonstrated extensively in Chapter 6, the score adjustment facility of a MFRM analysis provides linear measures of examinee proficiency corrected for the severity of the particular raters each examinee encountered in the assessment procedure.

Third, G-theory emphasizes rater homogeneity with a goal of making raters function interchangeably, whereas MFRM encourages rater self-consistency and expects raters to disagree with each other to some extent. These differences in focus imply different conceptions of what constitutes an "ideal rater". According to

---

17 This G-theory analysis was based on a *random-effects model*; that is, raters and criteria were considered random samples from the universe. Alternatively, the criterion effect could be considered a fixed effect in a given D-study, in which case the investigator would not be interested in generalizing beyond the present criteria. Applying such a *mixed model* changed the results only slightly. For example, the generalizability coefficient for D-study 1 changed from .844 to .856, that for D-study 3 from .909 to .922.

G-theory, the ideal rater provides ratings freed from any errors and biases, using the rating scale in an identical manner under identical conditions. By contrast, the MFRM view is that the ideal rater acts as an independent expert, exhibiting a specific amount of leniency or severity, and using the rating scale in a consistent manner across examinees, criteria, etc. Within G-theory, between-rater severity differences are considered a source of measurement error that is to be minimized; proponents of a MFRM approach accept them as a critical part of ineradicable rater variability that calls for psychometric adjustment.

Though it is commonly acknowledged that G-theory and MFRM modeling represent markedly different approaches to the problem of measurement error, researchers have also pointed to some complementary utility (e.g., Iramaneerat et al., 2008; Kim & Wilson, 2009; Lynch & McNamara, 1998; Sudweeks et al., 2005). In particular, this refers to the *level of analysis* characterizing each approach: Whereas G-theory views the data largely from a group-level perspective, disentangling the sources of measurement error and estimating their magnitude, a MFRM analysis focuses more on individual-level information and thus promotes substantive investigation into the behavior, or functioning, of each individual element of the facets under consideration.

Hence, depending on the purpose of the assessment there may be some merit in combining both approaches. As Kim and Wilson (2009) put it:

> If it is important to estimate the similarity between the observed raw scores of the group of students and the raw scores that similar groups of students might obtain under identical circumstances, G theory may be helpful. If it is important to estimate for each student a measure as free as possible of the particularities of the facets that generated the raw score, then MFRM is highly desirable. (p. 422)

9.5 MFRM software and extensions

Throughout this book, MFRM analyses were conducted by means of the computer program FACETS (Version 3.71; Linacre, 2014a). Over the years, FACETS has gained great popularity among Rasch practitioners working in a wide range of applied fields. FACETS is a highly versatile program that provides users with lots of MFRM model instantiations, analytical tools, and statistical indicators, and it offers a host of flexible input and output functions, reporting measurement results in user-specified tables and graphical displays. At the website http://www.winsteps.com, interested readers will find detailed information on the program and the Rasch models it implements, as well as a set of four highly instructive FACETS tutorial PDFs. Also, the FACETS manual (Linacre, 2014b) is available at the website as a free download; this manual contains many illustrative examples of FACETS specifications and data analyses as well as explanations of measurement output tables and graphs. Moreover, the website offers a free student/evaluation version called MINIFAC.

There are a number of other computer programs that can be used to conduct MFRM analyses, including ConQuest (Adams, Wu, & Wilson, 2012), RUMM (Andrich, Sheridan, & Luo, 2010), IRTPRO (Cai, Thissen, & du Toit, 2013), and LPCM-WIN (Fischer & Ponocny-Seliger, 2003). With respect to R, the free software environment for statistical computing and graphics (R Core Team, 2014), several packages are available that allow implementing, among other things, many-facet Rasch models, such as eRm (Extended Rasch Modeling; Mair, Hatzinger, & Maier, 2014; see also Mair & Hatzinger, 2007a, 2007b), sirt (Supplementary Item Response Theory Models; Robitzsch, 2014), and TAM (Test Analysis Modules; Kiefer, Robitzsch, & Wu, 2014).

The aformentioned programs differ in many respects, including the statistical techniques they employ for estimating model parameters. Most often, one of the following techniques is used: joint maximum likelihood (FACETS, sirt, TAM), marginal maximum likelihood (ConQuest, IRTPRO), pairwise conditional (RUMM), and conditional maximum likelihood (LPCM-WIN, eRm). Note that sirt and TAM additionally employ marginal maximum likelihood techniques.

There has been a theoretical debate about the relative merits of each technique (e.g., Baker & Kim, 2004; Linacre, 2004a, 2004c; Molenaar, 1995; Verhelst, 2004). In particular, joint maximum likelihood estimation has been criticized for its lack of consistency (Cohen, Chan, Jiang, & Seburn, 2008; Molenaar, 1995). However, some authors suggested that the differences in the estimates produced by each of these techniques can be considered negligibly small for most practical purposes (Baker & Kim, 2004; Linacre, 2004a; see also Kline et al., 2006).

Concerning the generality of the underlying measurement approach, ConQuest stands out by using one highly general model to fit a wide variety of Rasch models: the *multidimensional random coefficients multinomial logit model* (MRCMLM; Adams, Wilson, & Wang, 1997; see also Adams & Wu, 2007). An appealing feature of ConQuest is the option to perform *hierarchical model testing*. Choosing this option allows the investigator to systematically compare competing models that may each be considered appropriate for the data given. For example, let Model A specify examinees, criteria, raters, and an examinee-by-rater interaction. This model may be compared to a more parsimonious Model B (i.e., a submodel of A), created by removing the interaction term from Model A. Significantly better fit of Model A would indicate that the interaction between examinees and raters is a source of variation in the ratings that is not to be ignored.

Another important feature of ConQuest refers to the option to implement *multidimensional* Rasch models. As mentioned earlier (see Section 8.2), such models may be called for when it is reasonable to assume that there are two or more latent proficiency dimensions simultaneously addressed by a test or an assessment. Furthermore, ConQuest's multidimensional option allows researchers to model local item dependence (LID). For example, LID may occur among a set of criteria on which raters provide ratings of examinee performance (Wang & Wilson, 2005a, 2005b). Multidimensional Rasch models can also be implemented through software packages like IRTPRO (Cai et al., 2013) or MULTIRA (Carstensen & Rost, 2003; see also Rost & Carstensen, 2002).

Finally, Muckle and Karabatsos (2009) have shown that the many-facet Rasch model can be considered a special case of the two-level hierarchical generalized linear model (HGLM). More generally, adopting a *multilevel* Rasch measurement perspective makes possible a number of extensions regarding the analysis of many-facet data, for example, modeling nested data structures, modeling longitudinal data, or modeling covariates of examinee proficiency, task difficulty, and rater severity (Dobria, 2011, 2012; Hung & Wang, 2012; Jiao, Wang, & Kamata, 2007; Kamata & Cheong, 2007). HGLMs can be implemented using software such as HLM 7 (Raudenbush, Bryk, Cheong, Congdon, & du Toit, 2011) or the lme4 package (Doran, Bates, Bliese, & Dowling, 2007; Bates et al., 2014; see also Lamprianou, 2013). Roberts and Herrington (2007) demonstrated the use of different HGLM measurement programs.

10. Summary and Conclusions

This final chapter provides a look back on critical concepts and issues of the MFRM approach to the analysis and evaluation of rater-mediated assessments. The first section reconsiders major steps and procedures and presents a summary in a flowchart-like diagram. Throughout the book, a single data set drawn from a writing assessment program was used for illustrative purposes. To broaden the perspective and to underscore the versatility of the MFRM approach, the second section briefly discusses MFRM studies in diverse fields of application, ranging from psychological assessment to medical education and occupational behavior. A major theme of the book has been that conducting a MFRM analysis strongly contributes to ensuring the validity and fairness of interpretations and uses of assessment outcomes. In two separate sections, this theme is explored more deeply.

10.1 Major steps and procedures

Chapter 1 introduced the basic three-step measurement approach to rater-mediated assessments: Identifying potentially relevant facets, specifying an appropriate measurement model, and applying this model to the assessment data. In this section, I elaborate on this approach. Building on a sequence of seven more detailed steps, I review relevant concepts, procedures, and model implementations discussed in the previous chapters. Figure 10.1 presents these steps in a diagrammatic form. Within each box representing a given step, a short list of keywords is provided that illustrate concepts, issues, and procedures typically involved in that step. Arrows between the boxes indicate the usual sequence of steps, which may be altered depending on the assessment or research context.

Fig. 10.1: A seven-step measurement approach to the analysis and evaluation of rater-mediated assessments.

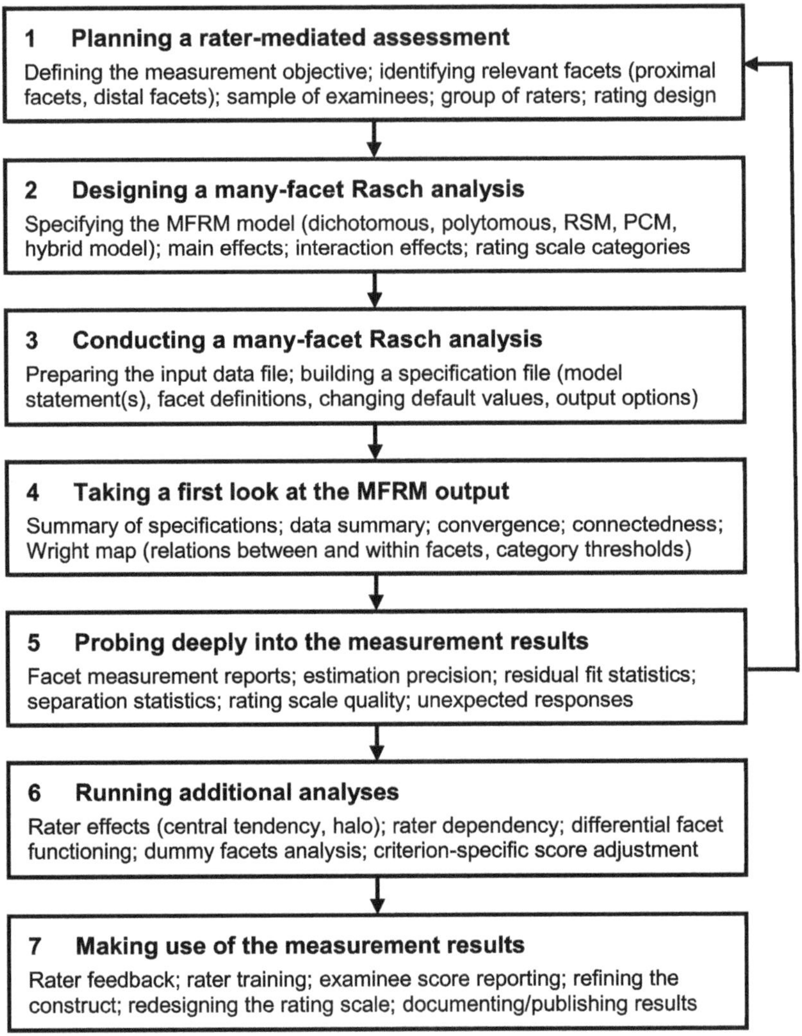

Any rater-mediated assessment that aims at conducting a MFRM analysis must start with a precise definition of the measurement objective. This definition should take into account the broader assessment context (e.g., low-stakes or high-stakes assessment, time and budget constraints, availability of rater training and monitoring opportunities), the nature of the performances or products to be evaluated, and the specifics of the assessment instrument, including the number and kind of performance tasks (e.g., limited production tasks like short-answer questions or extended production tasks like essay writing prompts), the scoring criteria, and the scoring rubric. In keeping with the conceptual–psychometric framework outlined in Section 3.3, the planning phase basically consists of identifying the proximal and distal facets that are likely to contribute to the assessment outcomes. In particular, key questions refer to the sample of examinees at which the assessment is targeted, the group of sufficiently qualified raters, and the plan for assigning raters to examinees, tasks, or criteria. Choosing a suitable rating design has direct consequences for the connectedness of the resulting data matrix (see Step 4 below).

After its completion, the planning phase should provide the pieces of information needed to specify the measurement model (Step 2). Thus, it should be clear whether the input data conform to a dichotomous (correct/incorrect, yes/no, pass/fail) or a polytomous format (three or more qualitatively ordered categories) or a mixture of both formats, or even some other format (e.g., binomial trials). Depending on extant information about the scoring format, differences in raters' rating style, and the number or responses that can be used for estimation, various instantiations of the many-facet Rasch model may be specified, including the rating scale model, the partical credit model, or some hybrid model. At this stage of the analysis, the focus is on studying main effects and, possibly, interactions between those facets that were identified as proximal facets in the previous step.

The model designing phase is largely independent of the computer software used to implement a given MFRM model. Of course, this independence no longer holds true when it comes to conducting a MFRM analysis (Step 3). In the present book, I almost exclusively made reference to the FACETS program (Linacre, 2014a). This program accepts a wide range of differently formatted data files, and it also comes with a separate data formatter (FACFORM; Linacre, 2009) for use with highly complex or otherwise difficult-to-format data.

Once the data have been prepared for input into FACETS, the specification file is constructed. This file contains a set of instructions (commands) on how to analyze the data. Key commands refer to the model statement, the definition of the facets, and the choice among a large number of output options. Note that more than a single model statement may be included in the specifications, allowing different data formats or parts of the data set to be analyzed within the same frame of reference. For example, one subset of items may be scored dichotomously, another subset may have a rating scale structure, still another subset may have a partial credit structure. When using multiple model statements, the sequence of the statements is important; that is, FACETS attempts to match each data line to each model statement in turn, beginning with the first statement. The facet definitions include specifying the positive or negative scale orientation of the facets (where "positive" means "higher measure, higher score" and "negative" means "higher measure, lower score"), determining the facets to be centered in order to set the origin of the measurement scale, and the labeling of facets and their elements.

When looking at the FACETS output it is important to first make sure that the data were processed as expected (Step 4). Table 1 of the output provides a summary of the specifications that were used in the analysis. This summary should be inspected closely regarding the facet definitions as understood by the program, the model statements, and the warning messages (if any). Next, Table 2 of the output file presents a summary of the input data. For example, this table gives the number of responses matched to a particular model specified in the model statement and the number of valid responses used for estimation. These numbers should be checked for correctness before proceeding any further.

Table 3 of the FACETS output reports on the iteration process. The number of iterations performed is controlled by two commands: (a) the maximum number of iterations ("Iterations="), where the default value "0" permits an unlimited number of iterations, and (b) convergence criteria ("Convergence="), where the default values are ".5" (maximum size of the difference between observed and expected "total" raw scores after omission of extreme scores for any element) and ".01" (maximum size of the largest logit change in any estimated measure for an element during the previous iteration). When the convergence criteria are satisfied, the iteration process stops. In addition, during the iteration process the input data set is checked for connectedness, the prerequisite condition for constructing measures for the elements of all facets within the same frame of reference. If the data set proves to be connected, Table 3 reports "Subset connection O.K." after the last iteration; if it is not, a warning message appears such as "There may be 2 disjoint subsets" (for options to remedy the problem of disjoint subsets, see Section 9.1).

When the specifications were all correct, the input data were processed accordingly, and the estimation process converged with proof of connectedness, the next step is to look at the Wright map (Table 6 of the FACETS output). This map provides an invaluable source of information on the relations between and within the facets. Closely studying the map helps to gain first insights into a number of relevant assessment issues such as the following: What is the spread of the rater severity measures (compared to the spread of the examinee ability measures), what is the degree of the examinee-task or examinee-item alignment, that is, were the tasks or items designed in such a way that their difficulties matched examinee abilities, or what is the spacing of the category thresholds along the rating scale, that is, were the rating scale categories used as intended?

In a series of similarly organized tables, FACETS output presents detailed measurement results for each facet defined previously. Tables 5.1, 6.1, and 7.1 of the present book each reflect most (or part) of the information contained in the FACETS rater, examinee, and criterion measurement reports for the sample data analysis. These measurement reports provide information on the size of the parameter estimates, the estimates' precision, infit and outfit statistics, and fair averages. Probing deeply into the measurement reports (Step 5) is crucial for developing an understanding of the very nature of the assessment, its possible strengths and weaknesses. For example, unacceptably high values of the infit and outfit statistics often indicate that the assessment has failed to yield sufficiently meaningful measures, and they suggest where to look in the data to locate the problems. Fair averages show what the rater severity measures look like in the raw-score metric. In many instances, fair averages impressively demonstrate to lay audiences the extent to which raters' judgments of examinee performances differ when differences in examinee ability are taken into account. Each FACETS measurement report is completed by population and sample versions of separation statistics, including the separation ratio, the separation (strata) index, and the separation reliability.

Two more tables of the FACETS output provide important input to the evaluation of the assessment in Step 5: The scale category statistics (Table 7.3, this book), and the list of unexpected responses (Table 4.3, this book). The category statistics indicate whether the rating scale functioned as intended or whether it was deficient in some respect. Using the guidelines presented in Table 7.2 (this book) most of the problems in rating scale functioning may be diagnosed efficiently. For example, severe problems are indicated by reversed average measures by category or disordered category thresholds. The list of unexpected responses is controlled by the command "Unexpected=" in the specification file. For example, to let FACETS list all responses for which the absolute value of the standardized residuals is greater than or equal to 2.0, the command becomes "Unexpected=2" (the default value is "3"). Unexpected responses may come about for quite many reasons, such as incorrect formatting of data, use of an incorrect scoring key, or reversed rating scales. When there are patterns of unexpected responses, as when the same rater, examinee, or criterion appears in the listing many times, this is an indication of local misfit that should be studied carefully. Note that local misfit may not affect the summary fit statistics when it is concentrated on a small subset of elements. The "Usort=" command in FACETS helps to identify patterns of misfitting ratings associated with individual raters, examinees, criteria, etc. Inserting this flexible command into the specification file allows the researcher, for example, to sort observed scores, standardized residuals, or absolute values of standardized residuals by facets and size (in ascending or descending order).

When there is evidence of substantial misfit that cannot be resolved simply by reformatting the data, combining or reversing scale categories or the like, it may be advisable to return to Step 1 and reconsider the assessment design, possibly revising the assessment instrument, or reconstructing the rating plan to provide for stronger links between facet elements. Of course, this would necessitate a new round of data gathering and analysis, continuing with Step 2. When the major purpose of applying the MFRM modeling approach is to learn more about the various components of the assessment procedure, as would be the case in a research context, another option is to run additional analyses, as described in the next step.

The facet measurement results can be used as input to more detailed computations and analyses, focusing on each facet in turn, and possibly running analyses to look at the interaction between facets and at other more complex relations within the data (Step 6). Regarding the rater facet, residual fit and scale category statistics provide information on the presence of rater effects such as central tendency and halo, both at the group level and at the level of individual raters. Inserting the command "Inter-rater=x" into the specification file, where "x" is the number of the rater facet, yields the information needed to compute the Rasch-kappa index. This index allows to assess the extent to which raters functioned as independent experts or were striving for perfect interrater reliability.

Another instance of more detailed analyses refers to the study of differential facet functioning (DFF), that is, the exploratory or confirmatory study of facet interactions. If a researcher is solely interested in studying interactions between facets, leaving out of account main effects of particular facets, dummy facets may be introduced into the model specification. Most often, these facets represent categorical variables of examinees, raters, or the assessment situation. For example, specifying examinee gender as a dummy facet allows to study differential rater functioning related to examinee gender (i.e., gender-related rater bias). When preparing reports on examinee scores adjusted for rater severity, an informative way to do so is to adjust scores also at the level of individual scoring criteria, as described in some detail in Section 6.4.

Finally, in Step 7, the major issue concerns applying the measurement results to assessment design and practice. One option is to provide detailed feedback to raters and inform rater training activities. Though research has documented that rater effects are often highly resistent to change, rater training may help to reduce severity or leniency extremes, thus increasing the rater-examinee or rater-task alignment, and to improve the consistency of individual raters. Score reporting that builds on adjusted, fair scores, possibly including criterion-related score profiles, is of course one of the most important practical uses of MFRM results.

On a more theoretical note, the construction of linear measures from qualitatively ordered observations provides a suitable basis for refining the assessment instrument and the conceptualization of the latent variable being assessed, for changing the design of the rating scale, or for rethinking the population of examinees at which the assessment is targeted. Considering the time and effort that is usually put into planning and performing rater-mediated assessments and running MFRM analyses, and with a view to the implications of measurement results for examinees and other stakeholders, particularly in high-stakes settings, it almost goes without saying that the assessment procedure and the measurement results should be communicated appropriately to a wider audience. As an aside, documenting and publishing measurement results helps to disseminate the rationale and practical utility of the MFRM approach to rater-mediated assessments.

10.2 MFRM across the disciplines

Throughout the book, I referred to the same three-facet data set containing scores that 18 raters awarded to the writing performance of 307 examinees; this group of raters provided ratings on each of three criteria using a four-category rating scale. For the purposes of this introductory text, the focus on a single connecting example allowed to gradually develop the basic principles, concepts, and analytic procedures of many-facet Rasch measurement, leaving largely constant the assessment context, the subject matter, and the terminology. This also implied some degree of redundancy, with the intent to facilitate the reader's understanding of each chapter's new material.

On the other hand, focusing on a single data set makes it difficult to convey an adequate understanding of the broad range of applications in which many-facet Rasch measurement is employed to answer substantive questions. To be sure, from its very beginning, the MFRM approach has played a prominent role within the field of language testing and assessment (Linacre, 2011; McNamara & Knoch, 2012). Yet, as mentioned earlier, it has increasingly been adopted in highly varied disciplines and fields of research. A quick impression of the versatility of the MFRM approach is provided by perusing the list of references in Chapter 4 of the FACETS manual (Linacre, 2014b), which contains over 350 published MFRM studies. Moreover, in Chapter 7, that manual presents 18 worked out examples of MFRM specifications and data from widely differing fields of application. The widespread use of MFRM models across many disciplines can also be seen from inserting the keyword "many-facet Rasch" in the search field of an Internet search engine. As of May 2015, this search yielded some 50,000 results (about half as many for "multi-facet Rasch").

For the purposes of illustration, Table 10.1 presents a selection of 12 exemplary MFRM studies from seven different fields of application, covering a period of 25 years. In fact, Study 10 (Lunz, Wright, & Linacre, 1990) was among the first MFRM studies ever. In Table 10.1, the studies are listed in alphabetical order of the references (last column). For each study, the table briefly notes the major research objective, the various facets considered (examinees, raters, and any additional facets), and two kinds of separation statistics, that is, the rater separation index (H) and the rater separation reliability (R). Four studies did not report the rater separation index. In these cases, I computed H from R using the transformation $G = \sqrt{(R(1 - R))}$, and inserted the resulting value of G into Formula 4.8 (Section 4.3).

The elements rated were in most cases examinees, in others the elements were test items, product samples, three-person teams, or the like. As can be seen, their number varied greatly from 3 elements (Study 11) to 8,642 elements (Study 5, a genuine large-scale assessment). Two studies did not employ raters as a separate group (Studies 2 and 4), and, thus, in a strict sense of the term, would not count as rater-mediated assessments; yet, in these cases, ratings (or judgments) were provided by participants within the context of a psychological study. The number of raters in the remaining ten studies ranged from 3 raters (Study 7) to 605 raters (Study 5).

Most studies employed a three-facet design, the others employed a two- or four-facet design. When reported, the rater homogeneity index Q was highly significant in each and every study ($p < .01$). Importantly, the rater separation (strata) index H ranged from 2.43 (Study 5) to 11.45 (Study 3), indicating that in not a single study raters (or participants) functioned interchangeably, that is, raters did not exhibit similar degrees of severity or leniency; much the same basic information is conveyed by the rater separation reliability, taking on values around .90 or higher in the majority of studies. As repeatedly noted throughout this book, rater heterogeneity is the rule rather than the exception.

Table 10.1: Illustrative MFRM Studies in Different Fields of Application: Research Objectives, Facets, and Separation Statistics.

Study No.	Field of Application	Research Objective	*N*	*J*	Other Facets	*H*	*R*	Reference
1	Educational Assessment	Evaluating the alignment of items to content standards	1,345	15	–	9.17[a]	.98[a]	Anderson, Irvin, Alonzo, and Tindal (2015)
2	Psychological Assessment	Studying implicit prejudice toward black people	880[b]	–	Conditions (2), Stimuli (28)	4.19	.94	Anselmi, Vianello, and Robusto (2011)
3	Language Assessment	Measuring speaking ability through group oral testing	1,324	20	Criteria (5)	11.45	.99	Bonk and Ockey (2003)
4	Psychological Assessment	Measuring persons' self-talk tendency	1,051[c]	–	Items (16), Subscales (4)	4.72	.92	Brinthaupt and Kang (2014)
5	Educational Assessment	Evaluating AP ELC performance assessment	8,642	605	Tasks (3)	2.43	.71	Engelhard and Myford (2003)
6	Medical Education	Measuring physician–patient communication skills	190	67	Cases (7), Items (28)	4.57[d]	.91	Harasym, Woloschuk, and Cunning (2008)
7	Language Assessment	Analyzing rater effects in Japanese writing assessment	234	3	Criteria (5)	9.67[d]	.98	Kondo-Brown (2002)
8	Physical Education	Evaluating judgments at the 2010 Olympic figure skating	24	9	Program components (5)	2.84[d]	.78	Looney (2012)
9	Consumer Behavior	Assessing the quality of product samples	6	43	Attributes (2), Time periods (4)	4.09	.89	Lunz and Linacre (1998)
10	Medical Education	Measuring performance on clinical examinations	217	18	Histology slides (15)	6.07	.95	Lunz, Wright, and Linacre (1990)

Study No.	Field of Application	Research Objective	N	J	Other Facets	H	R	Reference
11	Occupational Behavior	Evaluating pilot instructor rater training	3[e]	33	Criteria (12)	2.77[d]	.77	Mulqueen, Baker, and Dismukes (2002)
12	Medical Education	Evaluating student selection using the MMI	452	156	Stations (10), Examiner groups (3)	4.11	.89	Till, Myford, and Dowell (2013)

Note. N = number of examinees (or other elements being rated). J = number of raters. H = rater separation (strata) index. R = rater separation reliability. AP ELC = Advanced Placement English Literature and Composition. MMI = Multiple Mini-Interview. [a]D. Anderson, personal communication, October 17, 2014 (no separation statistics reported in the original study). [b]Respondents categorized stimuli presented on a computer screen as quickly as possible. [c]Respondents indicated frequency of self-talk on a five-category rating scale. [d]H value computed from the tabulated R value (H was not reported in the original study). [e]Pilot instructors rated the performance of complete cockpit crews (captain, first officer, and flight engineer).

Clearly, it is beyond the scope of this section to discuss the studies listed in Table 10.1 in any detail. Yet, to highlight the practical relevance and utility of the MFRM approach, three studies shall be examined somewhat more closely (i.e., Studies 1, 11, and 12).

In Study 1 (Anderson, Irvin, Alonzo, & Tindal, 2015), the research objective was to assess the alignment of test items to content standards. Fifteen middle school math teachers rated the degree to which content in math items, which covered Grades 6 to 8, matched the content in the standards they were intended to measure. Using a four-category scale (0 = *no alignment*, 1 = *vague alignment*, 2 = *somewhat aligned*, 3 = *directly aligned*), each teacher rated the alignment of approximately 270 items; each item was rated by three teachers (the total number of items was 1,345).

Building on a two-facet RSM, the researchers analyzed the alignment of items and the severity of raters. To determine whether an item did or did not align with the corresponding standard, the adjusted (or fair) item averages were employed. Only items having values as great or greater than 2.0 were classified as "aligned"; that is, these items were deemed appropriate for inclusion in operational test forms. Similarly, fair rater averages were employed to examine the degree to which raters differed from one another in their views of item alignment. Results showed that on average the most severe rater rated items 1.38 raw-score points lower than the most lenient rater—a difference that is not only statistically, but also practically highly significant.

Study 11 (Mulqueen, Baker, & Dismukes, 2002) was concerned with examining the effectiveness of pilot instructor rater training. Usually, after extensive training sessions, including line operational simulation (LOS) scenarios, pilot instructors' ratings of technical and crew resource management (CRM) skills are used to determine whether or not each pilot in the crew should be certified to fly the line. LOS scenarios involve a complete cockpit crew (e.g., captain, first officer, and flight engineer) performing on event sets in a realistic high-fidelity flight simulator. In the study, thirty-three pilot instructors first rated the videotaped performance of two different crews on the same three scenario events, where Crew 1 demonstrated average performance and Crew 2 demonstrated low performance. Based on these ratings, a consensus index of interrater reliability was computed (i.e., the within-group interrater agreement index, r_{wg}; James, Demaree, & Wolf, 1984, 1993); the results of this and further descriptive analyses were fed back to the group of raters. Then, pilot instructors rated the videotaped performance of a third crew flying the same scenario events, demonstrating high performance. In each case, ratings were provided using a four-category scale (1 = *repeat*, 2 = *debrief*, 3 = *standard*, 4 = *excellent*).

The average interrater agreement (r_{wg}) values for Crews 1, 2, and 3 were .70, .58, and .78, respectively. At first sight, these values indicated moderate to high agreement. However, the three-facet RSM analysis portrayed a completely different picture: As judged by the separation statistics, $R_J = .77$, $Q_J = 150.8$ ($df = 32$, $p < .01$), pilot instructors strongly disagreed with one another regarding their views of the crews' technical and CRM skills. Moreover, an analysis of the interaction between pilot instructors and crews revealed that some instructors even held opposing views on the performance of Crews 2 and 3. Mulqueen et al. (2002) reached the following conclusion: "If it were acceptable to the air carrier involved, an adjustment to pilot instructors' total scores for specified crews could be made based on the results of these analyses" (p. 300). Considering the vital importance of accurate ratings of crew performance, it may be advisable to implement such adjustments on a routine basis.

In Study 12 (Till, Myford, & Dowell, 2013), the focus was on investigating the usefulness of the multiple mini-interview (MMI) as an instrument to select candidates for entry into medical school. The MMI builds on the format of the objective structured clinical examination (OSCE); that is, the MMI consists of a series of stations in which examiners rate each candidate on six personal attributes (or domains) that medical schools value: interpersonal skills and communication (including empathy), logical reasoning and critical thinking, moral and ethical reasoning, motivation and preparation to study medicine, teamwork and leadership, and honesty and integrity (Eva, Rosenfeld, Reiter, & Norman, 2004). In the MMI considered here, a total of 156 examiners rated 452 candidates using a five-category scale (1 = *extremely poor*, 2 = *poor*, 3 = *adequate*, 4 = *good*, 5 = *ideal*). Based on their raw scores computed from these ratings, the candidates were ranked; medical school places were offered to the top-ranked 319 candidates.

At each station, a single examiner rated each candidate's performance. In order to ensure connectedness of the data, the rating design required examiners to participate in at least two half-day sessions of the MMI and in different stations. Thus, the design was incomplete but connected, allowing measures of candidate ability, examiner severity, and station difficulty to be reported on one common scale.

Employing a three-facet RSM, Till et al. (2013) found that the candidate separation reliability was .89 and the separation index was 4.07. This suggested that there were about four statistically distinct levels of ability in the candidate sample. So far, so good. But the values of the separation statistics for the examiner facet were much the same: the examiner separation reliability was .89, with a separation index of 4.11. That is, there were about four statistically distinct levels of severity in the group of examiners. The implication of this last finding is clear: Because different subsets of examiners rated each candidate, a given candidate's position in the ranking, based on raw score totals, would also depend on the ratio of severe to lenient examiners that happened to be included in the subset of examiners rating that candidate.

To illustrate the effect of compensating for between-rater severity differences, Till et al. (2013) compared the candidate ranking actually used in the MMI selection process with a ranking based on fair scores. Building on the fair score ranking, the selection outcomes would have changed for no less than 43 candidates (9.6% of the candidate sample). As summarized by Till et al. (2013, p. 216), "the analyses highlighted the fact that quality control monitoring is essential to ensure fairness when ranking candidates according to scores obtained in the MMI", leading the researchers to conclude that "'fair average' scores should be used for ranking the candidates" (p. 216).

10.3 Measurement and validation

The example of MMI selection decisions clearly demonstrates the critical importance of employing a MFRM-based score adjustment approach: In the Till et al. (2013) study, the logit range of rater severities was about two-third of the logit range of candidate abilities. Thus, chances were that the *most able* candidate and the *least able* candidate would have achieved the *same* raw score total (and, as a result, highly similar ranking positions), if the first one had happened to be rated by highly severe raters, and the second one had happened to be rated by highly lenient raters. An earlier MMI evaluation study adopting a similar MFRM approach (Roberts, Rothnie, Zoanetti, & Crossley, 2010) reported an equally high rater separation reliability (R_J = .91) and confirmed the strong impact of rater severity measures on candidate rankings.

Within the context of a speaking assessment, Coniam (2008) noted that the "issue of raw scores and consequent disparity of results through rater severity is one which merits substantial consideration" (p. 188). Even more emphatically, Bonk and Ockey (2003; see Table 10.1, Study 3) pointed out that neglecting to control for severity effects "would be irresponsible and may lead to spurious interpretations and/or decisions" (p. 104).

On a more general note, measuring rater severity and studying rater severity effects have an important role to play in establishing the fairness and validity of interpretations and uses of assessment outcomes. Viewed from this perspective, Steps 1 through 7 of a standard MFRM study (see Figure 10.1) can be interpreted as a systematic approach to providing validity evidence needed for the evaluation of rater-mediated assessments. To be sure, the concepts of validity and validation are themselves multi-faceted and have been the subject of much recent debate (e.g., Lissitz, 2009; Markus & Borsboom, 2013; Newton & Shaw, 2014). Hence, in what follows I only briefly deal with these concepts as they relate to a measurement approach to the evaluation of performance assessments (for a related discussion of measure validation using Rasch models, see Wolfe & Smith, 2007a, 2007b; see also Aryadoust, 2009).

According to the *argument-based framework* (Kane, 1992, 2006, 2013), validation has two components: (a) specification of the proposed interpretations and uses of test scores (the interpretation/use argument, IUA), and (b) evaluation of the plausibility of the proposed interpretations and uses (the validity argument). In line with this framework, the *Standards for Educational and Psychological Testing* (American Educational Research Association et al., 2014) pointed out that "it is the interpretations of test scores for proposed uses that are evaluated, not the test itself" (p. 11). Building validity arguments for rater-mediated assessments involves, first, stating propositions (or claims) about the raters' behavior and the quality of their ratings, and, second, collecting evidence to evaluate the soundness of each proposition, that is, to determine to what extent the evidence supports (or refutes) the proposed score interpretations (Kane, 2013).

The *Standards* underscored the importance of studying not only the response processes of examinees (test takers), but also the response processes of raters (observers, judges): "Assessments often rely on observers or judges to record and/ or evaluate test takers' performances or products. In such cases, relevant validity evidence includes the extent to which the processes of observers or judges are consistent with the intended interpretation of scores" (American Educational Research Association et al., 2014, p. 15). Response processes of raters that are inconsistent with the intended score interpretations (propositions) have been dealt with in this book in terms of factors contributing to construct-irrelevant variance in ratings (e.g., various forms of rater bias; Section 3.1).

Using the MMI as an example, Till, Myford, and Dowell (2015) developed propositions and examined various sources of rater-related validity evidence. Till et al. posed a set of rater-related propositions and associated research questions. Answering these questions was to help evaluate the propositions as required for building a validity argument. Empirical evidence for each proposition was provided by the MFRM analysis of the MMI rating data described previously (Till et al., 2013).

To illustrate, one of the propositions referred to the level of rater severity. The critical part of this proposition read as follows (note that Till et al. considered three groups of examiners; i.e., staff members, senior medical students, and simulated patients): "Within each examiner group, the examiners exercise similar levels of severity when rating candidates' personal attributes; it does not matter which particular examiner within that group rates which particular candidate." (Till et al., 2015, p. 11).

The research question associated with this proposition was: "Within each examiner group, did the examiners differ in the severity with which they rated candidates' personal attributes? If they did differ in severity, how did those differences affect candidates' scores and the selection outcomes?" (Till et al., 2015, p. 11).

The MFRM-based evidence regarding this question was clear: While the three rater groups did not differ significantly from one another in terms of average severity measures, *within* each group there were pronounced rater severity differences (the rater separation reliability ranged from .88 to .91); importantly, these severity differences had a demonstrable impact on the final candidate rankings. Therefore, Till et al. (2015) reached the following judgment: "This proposition does not seem sound, and the evidence gathered does not appear to support the proposed score interpretation" (p. 22). The ensuing recommendation that the medical school should consider using candidates' "fair average" measures rather than their raw score totals to rank order candidates has already been addressed above.

In a related study, Till, Ker, Myford, Stirling, and Mires (2015) constructed and evaluated a validity argument for the final-year Ward Simulation Exercise (FYWSE), designed to assist in determining whether senior medical students have acquired the level of clinical ability needed to provide high quality patient care. Using both MFRM and G-theory approaches, Till, Ker, et al. (2015) found that differences in examiner severity were not as pronounced as they were in the MMI validation study. Yet, the examiners were not interchangeable, leading again to unfairness in the final outcomes for some medical students.

As mentioned earlier (Section 3.1), the traditional approach to address differences in rater severity and other sources of rater variability does not follow this detailed, measurement-based validation process. Rather, the traditional approach rests on (a) having two or more raters evaluate the same performance, (b) resolving any critical rater disagreements by means of a defined procedure, and (c) computing an index of interrater reliability with the aim of documenting high levels of rating accuracy.

One of the practical problems associated with the traditional approach concerns resolving rater disagreements in order to report a single score to each examinee. Several resolution methods have been proposed, such as averaging the two original scores ("rater mean"), incorporating the rating of a third rater during adjudication ("parity method"), or replacing both original scores by the score of an expert adjudicator ("expert method"; e.g., Johnson et al., 2009; Johnson, Penny, Gordon, Shumate, & Fisher, 2005; Myford & Wolfe, 2002). In a simulation study (Penny & Johnson, 2011), the expert method outperformed the other methods, presupposing that the expert was indeed a highly proficient rater; otherwise, the parity method seemed to be well-suited (e.g., for purposes of research studies). However, it should be kept in mind that any of these methods builds on unadjusted, observed scores that may largely obscure the actual ability of the examinees or whatever the assessment intends to measure. Moreover, as highlighted by the agreement–accuracy paradox, low-validity or unfair ratings may go undetected when the raters involved exhibit much the same level of severity or leniency.

In view of the well-documented advantages of Rasch-based score adjustment, Lamprianou (2008) asked: "Why do a number of testing agencies and other exam-setting institutions around the world not use raw score adjustment methods?" (p. 85). Apart from obvious issues such as availability of appropriate computer programs and experience with program usage, the answer to this question is at least threefold: (a) Rasch-based score adjustment rests on a sophisticated statistical approach that is much more difficult to explain to a lay audience (teachers, parents, examinees, etc.) than any of the disagreement resolution methods, (b) employing a disagreement resolution method such as the expert method enhances the *face validity* of performance assessments, that is, such a method strengthens lay persons' beliefs in the accuracy of an assessment procedure, and (c) making use of Rasch-based score adjustment presupposes that the input data meet certain requirements, such as a network of links between facet elements (i.e., connectedness), a sufficiently large number of responses used for estimation, and a satisfactory data–model fit, particularly regarding within-rater consistency.

Ensuring within-rater consistency is indeed an important concern in score adjustments. Unless each rater has been shown to hold much the same level of severity or leniency across all examinees rated, that is, unless rater fit statistics have been shown to stay within reasonable limits, adjusting observed scores for between-rater severity differences can give rise to problems. When, for example, a particular rater exhibited pronounced leniency toward the majority of examinees but, for some reason or other, tended to severity toward a small subgroup of examinees, indiscriminate downward adjustment of scores would clearly be unfair to examinees in that subgroup.

One approach to attain sufficiently high consistency at the level of individual raters is through careful rater training along with regular monitoring activities. In particular, rater monitoring could be combined with detailed, diagnostic feedback based on rater measurement results. More advanced analyses may address various forms of rater bias or differential rater functioning, possibly complemented by specific rater retraining.

In case of multiple ratings of the same performance, another validity issue concerns the extent to which raters act as independent experts, as presupposed by adopting a MFRM approach, or provide ratings that in some way or other yield limited, redundant, or errant information. When, for example, an assessment program forces raters to agree with one another, penalizing raters in case of disagreements, the validity of score interpretations and uses may be threatened because the range of performance features raters consider in the process of rating is essentially restricted to those features that are assumed to boost interrater agreement and reliability.

In order to check whether the raters referred to their expert knowledge of the performance or proficiency domain under study, providing ratings independently of each other, or whether they tended to produce a level of agreement much higher than expected on the basis of the many-facet Rasch model, using the Rasch-kappa index (Linacre, 2014b; see Section 5.3) appears to be a viable option. Clearly, though, this index needs to be studied carefully in order to learn more about its statistical properties, its range of application, and its diagnostic value for various kinds of data.

More recently, researchers have developed psychometric approaches that are designed to explicitly model local rater dependence. These include the rater bundle model (Wilson & Hoskens, 2001), the hierarchical rater model (Patz et al., 2002; for a critique of this model, see Linacre, 2003a), the IRT model for multiple raters (Verhelst & Verstralen, 2001), the latent class signal detection rater model (DeCarlo, 2005; DeCarlo, Kim, & Johnson, 2011), and Yao's rater model (Wang & Yao, 2013).

The relative merits, prospects, and limitations of these and related modeling approaches need to be addressed more fully in future research. First steps in this direction have already been taken (e.g., Barr & Raju, 2003; Bock, Brennan, & Muraki, 2002; Guo, 2014; Mariano & Junker, 2007; Wang, Su, & Qiu, 2014; Wolfe & Song, 2014).

10.4 MFRM and the study of rater cognition

A recurring theme of this book has been the complex nature of the rating process. This process often places high cognitive demands on raters. Thus, raters have been described as perceiving, interpreting, and categorizing examinee responses, drawing on their expert knowledge, and integrating and retrieving memory information for judgment and decision making. A summary term for these and related mental activities that raters typically engage in is *rater cognition*. Generally speaking, rater cognition refers to the mental structures and processes involved in assigning ratings to examinee performances or products. In line with the rater cognition perspective, raters have been variously conceived of as *information processors* (Freedman & Calfee, 1983; Suto, 2012), *decision makers* (Baker, 2012; Cumming, Kantor, & Powers, 2002), or *social perceivers* (Govaerts, Van de Wiel, Schuwirth, Van der Vleuten, & Muijtjens, 2013).

Bejar (2012) characterized rater cognition as an emerging field of research with strong implications for the validity of inferences that are based on assessment outcomes. With reference to Kane's (1992, 2006) argument-based validation framework, Bejar pointed out that "rater cognition is central to a validity argument based on human scores" (p. 6). Similarly, Myford (2012) emphasized that "the collection and examination of evidence regarding the cognitive processes that raters employ is critical to validation efforts for rater-mediated assessments" (p. 48). Clearly, this kind of reasoning is reflected in the *Standards* (American Educational Research Association et al., 2014), where the degree of consistency of raters' response processes with the intended score interpretations is considered an important source of validity evidence.

The preceding section on measurement and validation showed that the MFRM approach has an important role to play in the collection and examination of validity evidence regarding rater-mediated assessments. Yet, this approach can only contribute a part to the overall validation work. In particular, MFRM models are not suited to specifically address raters' cognitive processes; that is, MFRM studies are well equipped to examine between-rater severity differences and rater biases, but they cannot reveal the basic judgmental or decision-making processes involved in assigning harsh, lenient, or overly inconsistent ratings. Therefore, in order to achieve a broader and deeper understanding of the human rating process it is necessary to complement or combine MFRM results with findings from research explicitly designed to study such processes. This can also help provide rich and varied empirical evidence required for building convincing validity arguments.

Researchers in the field of rater-mediated assessments have typically adopted either a quantitative approach, such as MFRM, G-theory, linear regression, and factor analysis (e.g., Lane & Stone, 2006; McNamara, 1996; Purpura, 2011), or a qualitative approach, including think-aloud reporting, discourse analysis, semi-structured interviews, retrospective written reports, and stimulated recall (e.g., Lazaraton, 2008; Sasaki, 2014; Suto, 2012). By comparison, qualitative approaches have the distinct advantage of allowing researchers to examine more process-oriented issues of assessments. For example, the analysis of think-aloud (or verbal) protocols is a method for collecting and analyzing verbal data about cognitive processing. This method involves making a detailed record of a person's verbal report while he or she is engaged in carrying out a task, such as reading an essay or assigning a score to a performance. Vaughan (1991) used think-alouds to answer the question of what goes on in a rater's mind during holistic assessment of writing performance. She identified a number of reading styles like the "first-impression-dominates style" or the "grammar-oriented style", concluding that raters focused on different essay elements and came to rely on an individual approach to reading essays. Cumming et al. (2002) similarly studied raters' cognitive processes and found that essay evaluation involved "interactive, multifaceted decision making" (p. 88). Adding to this line of research, Barkaoui (2010) showed that the rating scale had a larger effect on raters' decision-making behaviors than amount of rater experience (i.e., novice vs. experienced raters).

One of the major challenges facing the field today is combining quantitative and qualitative approaches in an efficient way and making informed choices regarding the particular methods to be used in a given research context (Myford, 2012; see also Lumley & Brown, 2005). The combination, or integration, of quantitative and qualitative methods in a single study has come to be called a *mixed methods* approach, or "the third research paradigm" (Turner, 2014, p. 1403). In principle, employing a mixed methods approach allows taking advantage of the strengths of the first two paradigms, while avoiding at least some of each paradigm's weaknesses or shortcomings (Creswell & Plano Clark, 2011).

In more recent years, researchers have begun to adopt a mixed methods approach to analyzing the rating process. For example, Kim (2009) investigated native and nonnative teachers' judgments of student performance on a semi-direct English speaking assessment. Teachers had to (a) assign ratings on a four-category scale and (b) justify their ratings by providing written reports or comments. A MFRM analysis of the rating data was combined with a frequency analysis of evaluation criteria extracted from the comments. Findings showed that teachers not only exercised different levels of severity but also drew on different evaluation criteria across speaking tasks. That is, teachers appeared to assign similar scores to the same performances but for somewhat different reasons. Yan (2014) used much the same mixed methods design focusing on implications for rater training (see also Carlsen, 2009).

The unique benefits offered by employing a mixed methods strategy have also been documented in research combining a MFRM approach with (a) raters' retrospective reports on their decision making collected through "write-aloud" protocols (Baker, 2012), (b) stimulated recall, where raters watched videos of themselves rating and explained their rating processes at the time of rating (Winke, Gass, & Myford, 2011), and (c) think-aloud tasks and follow-up interviews to gain insight into the meaningfulness of absolute magnitude estimation scales (Koskey & Stewart, 2014).

10.5 Concluding remarks

The strong interrelations that exist between the MFRM approach to rater-mediated assessments and the demands of ensuring the validity and fairness of interpretations and uses of assessment outcomes highlight the practical utility of many-facet Rasch models. Future methodological developments are likely to increase the utility and flexibility of Rasch measurement in complex assessment domains even further. Surely, this will also stimulate the study of basic and applied research issues in a large number of different disciplines and extend the already wide range of its application.

Over the years, MFRM has profoundly changed the way we think about rater-mediated assessment. It has changed the way we develop assessments, train and monitor raters, devise assessment procedures, including rating designs and rating scales, and, finally, construct and report measures of examinee proficiency or whatever the latent variable may be. Through illuminating the error-prone nature of human judgments and freeing assessment outcomes as much as possible from ubiquitous errors and biases, many-facet Rasch modeling offers a clear view of the object of measurement and thus advances our assessment knowledge, understandings, and practices.

The field of performance assessment has travelled a long and winding road to become part of the contemporary science of measurement. As a major contributor to this development, the many-facet Rasch model gets us from fallible, qualitatively ordered observations to linear measures that suitably represent an examinee's performance. Or, as Linacre (1989, p. 131) put it: "From the chaos of judge disagreement, the many-facet model brings the order of objective measurement".

References

Adams, R. J., Wilson, M., & Wang, W-C. (1997). The multidimensional random coefficients multinomial logit model. *Applied Psychological Measurement, 21,* 1–23.

Adams, R. J., & Wu, M. L. (2007). The mixed-coefficients multinomial logit model: A generalized form of the Rasch model. In M. von Davier & C. H. Carstensen (Eds.), *Multivariate and mixture distribution Rasch models: Extensions and applications* (pp. 57–75). New York, NY: Springer.

Adams, R., Wu, M., & Wilson, M. (2012). ConQuest (Version 3.0) [Computer software]. Camberwell, Australia: ACER Press.

Akiyama, T. (2001). The application of G-theory and IRT in the analysis of data from speaking tests administered in a classroom context. *Melbourne Papers in Language Testing, 10,* 1–21.

Alderson, J. C., & Banerjee, J. (2001). Language testing and assessment (Part 1). *Language Teaching, 34,* 213–236.

Alderson, J. C., & Banerjee, J. (2002). Language testing and assessment (Part 2). *Language Teaching, 35,* 79–113.

American Educational Research Association, American Psychological Association, & National Council on Measurement in Education. (2014). *Standards for educational and psychological testing.* Washington, DC: American Educational Research Association.

Andersen, E. B. (1982). Georg Rasch (1901–1980). *Psychometrika, 47,* 375–376.

Andersen, E. B. (2005). Rating scale model. *Encyclopedia of Social Measurement, 3,* 307–315.

Andersen, E. B., & Olsen, L. W. (2001). The life of Georg Rasch as a mathematician and as a statistician. In A. Boomsma, M. A. J. van Duijn, & T. A. B. Snijders (Eds.), *Essays on item response theory* (pp. 3–24). New York, NY: Springer.

Anderson, D., Irvin, P. S., Alonzo, J., & Tindal, G. A. (2015). Gauging item alignment through online systems while controlling for rater effects. *Educational Measurement: Issues and Practice, 34*(1), 22–33.

Andrich, D. (1978). A rating formulation for ordered response categories. *Psychometrika, 43,* 561–573.

Andrich, D. (1988). *Rasch models for measurement.* Newbury Park, CA: Sage.

Andrich, D. (1998). Thresholds, steps and rating scale conceptualization. *Rasch Measurement Transactions, 12,* 648–649.

Andrich, D. (2004). Controversy and the Rasch model: A characteristic of incompatible paradigms? *Medical Care, 42*(Supplement 1), I7–I16.

Andrich, D. (2005a). Rasch, Georg. *Encyclopedia of Social Measurement, 3*, 299–306.

Andrich, D. (2005b). Rasch models for ordered response categories. In B. S. Everitt & D. Howell (Eds.), *Encyclopedia of statistics in behavioral science* (Vol. 3, pp. 1698–1707). New York, NY: Wiley.

Andrich, D. (2010). Understanding the response structure and process in the polytomous Rasch model. In M. L. Nering & R. Ostini (Eds.), *Handbook of polytomous item response theory models* (pp. 123–152). New York, NY: Routledge.

Andrich, D., de Jong, J. H. A. L., & Sheridan, B. E. (1997). Diagnostic opportunities with the Rasch model for ordered response categories. In J. Rost & R. Langeheine (Eds.), *Applications of latent trait and latent class models in the social sciences* (pp. 59–72). Münster, Germany: Waxmann.

Andrich, D., Sheridan, B. E., & Luo, G. (2010). RUMM2030: Rasch unidimensional measurement models [Computer software]. Perth, Australia: RUMM Laboratory.

Angoff, W. H. (1971). Scales, norms, and equivalent scores. In R. L. Thorndike (Ed.), *Educational measurement* (2nd ed., pp. 508–600). Washington, DC: American Council on Education.

Anselmi, P., Vianello, M., & Robusto, E. (2011). Positive associations primacy in the IAT: A many-facet Rasch measurement analysis. *Experimental Psychology, 58*, 376–384.

Aryadoust, S. V. (2009). Mapping Rasch-based measurement onto the argument-based validity framework. *Rasch Measurement Transactions, 23*, 1192–1193.

Bachman, L. F. (2000). Modern language testing at the turn of the century: Assuring that what we count counts. *Language Testing, 17*, 1–42.

Bachman, L. F. (2002). Some reflections on task-based language performance assessment. *Language Testing, 19*, 453–476.

Bachman, L. F. (2004). *Statistical analyses for language assessment*. Cambridge, UK: Cambridge University Press.

Bachman, L. F., Lynch, B. K., & Mason, M. (1995). Investigating variability in tasks and rater judgements in a performance test of foreign language speaking. *Language Testing, 12*, 238–257.

Bachman, L. F., & Palmer, A. S. (1996). *Language testing in practice: Designing and developing useful language tests*. Oxford, UK: Oxford University Press.

Baghaei, P. (2007). Applying the Rasch rating-scale model to set multiple cut-offs. *Rasch Measurement Transactions, 20*, 1075–1076.

Baker, B. A. (2012). Individual differences in rater decision-making style: An exploratory mixed-methods study. *Language Assessment Quarterly, 9*, 225–248.

Baker, F. B., & Kim, S.-H. (2004). *Item response theory: Parameter estimation techniques* (2nd ed.). New York, NY: Dekker.

Barkaoui, K. (2010). Variability in ESL essay rating processes: The role of the rating scale and rater experience. *Language Assessment Quarterly, 7*, 54–74.

Barkaoui, K. (2014). Multifaceted Rasch analysis for test evaluation. In A. J. Kunnan (Ed.), *The companion to language assessment: Evaluation, methodology, and interdisciplinary themes* (Vol. 3, pp. 1301–1322). Chichester, UK: Wiley.

Barr, M. A., & Raju, N. S. (2003). IRT-based assessments of rater effects in multiple-source feedback instruments. *Organizational Research Methods, 6*, 15–43.

Barrett, S. (2001). The impact of training on rater variability. *International Education Journal, 2*, 49–58.

Barrett, S. (2005). Raters and examinations. In S. Alagumalai, D. C. Curtis & N. Hungi (Eds.), *Applied Rasch measurement: A book of exemplars – Papers in honour of John P. Keeves* (pp. 159–177). Dordrecht, The Netherlands: Springer.

Bates, D., Maechler, M., Bolker, B., Walker, S., Christensen, R. H. B., Singmann, H., & Dai, B. (2014). Package 'lme4' (Version 1.1–7) [Computer software and manual]. Retrieved from http://cran.R-project.org/web/packages/lme4/index.html

Bechger, T. M., Maris, G., & Hsiao, Y. P. (2010). Detecting halo effects in performance-based examinations. *Applied Psychological Measurement, 34*, 607–619.

Bejar, I. I. (1983). *Achievement testing: Recent advances.* Beverly Hills, CA: Sage.

Bejar, I. I. (2012). Rater cognition: Implications for validity. *Educational Measurement: Issues and Practice, 31*(3), 2–9.

Bejar, I. I., Williamson, D. M., & Mislevy, R. J. (2006). Human scoring. In D. M. Williamson, R. J. Mislevy, & I. I. Bejar (Eds.), *Automated scoring of complex tasks in computer-based testing* (pp. 49–81). Mahwah, NJ: Erlbaum.

Berry, V. (2007). *Personality differences and oral test performance.* Frankfurt, Germany: Lang.

Bock, R. D., Brennan, R. L., & Muraki, E. (2002). The information in multiple ratings. *Applied Psychological Measurement, 26*, 364–375.

Bond, T. G., & Fox, C. M. (2015). *Applying the Rasch model: Fundamental measurement in the human sciences* (3rd ed.). New York, NY: Routledge.

Bonk, W. J., & Ockey, G. J. (2003). A many-facet Rasch analysis of the second language group oral discussion task. *Language Testing, 20*, 89–110.

Boone, W. J., Staver, J. R., & Yale, M. S. (2014). *Rasch analysis in the human sciences.* Dordrecht, The Netherlands: Springer.

Boulet, J. R., & McKinley, D. W. (2005). Investigating gender-related construct-irrelevant components of scores on the written assessment exercise of a high-stakes certification assessment. *Advances in Health Sciences Education, 10,* 53–63.

Bramley, T. (2007). Quantifying marker agreement: Terminology, statistics and issues. *Research Matters: A Cambridge Assessment Publication, 4,* 22–28.

Brennan, R. L. (2001). *Generalizability theory.* New York, NY: Springer.

Brennan, R. L. (2011). Generalizability theory and classical test theory. *Applied Measurement in Education, 24,* 1–21.

Breton, G., Lepage, S., & North, B. (2008). *Cross-language benchmarking seminar to calibrate examples of spoken production in English, French, German, Italian and Spanish with regard to the six levels of the* Common European Framework of Reference for Languages (CEFR). Strasbourg, France: Council of Europe/ Language Policy Division.

Briggs, D. C., & Wilson, M. (2004). An introduction to multidimensional measurement using Rasch models. In E. V. Smith & R. M. Smith (Eds.), *Introduction to Rasch measurement* (pp. 322–341). Maple Grove, MN: JAM Press.

Brinthaupt, T. M., & Kang, M. (2014). Many-faceted Rasch calibration: An example using the Self-Talk Scale. *Assessment, 21,* 241–249.

Brown, A. (2005). *Interviewer variability in oral proficiency interviews.* Frankfurt, Germany: Lang.

Cai, L., Thissen, D., & du Toit, S. H. C. (2013). IRTPRO for Windows (Version 2.1) [Computer software]. Lincolnwood, IL: Scientific Software International.

Carlsen, C. (2009). *Guarding the guardians: Rating scale and rater training effects on test scores.* Saarbrücken, Germany: VDM.

Carr, N. T. (2011). *Designing and analyzing language tests.* Oxford, UK: Oxford University Press.

Carstensen, C. H., & Rost, J. (2003). MULTIRA: A program system for multidimensional Rasch models (Version 1.65) [Computer software]. Kiel, Germany: IPN—Leibniz Institute for Science Education.

Carstensen, C. H., & Rost, J. (2007). Multidimensional three-mode Rasch models. In M. von Davier & C. H. Carstensen (Eds.), *Multivariate and mixture distribution Rasch models: Extensions and applications* (pp. 157–175). New York, NY: Springer.

Chen, C.-T., & Wang, W.-C. (2007). Effects of ignoring item interaction on item parameter estimation and detection of interacting items. *Applied Psychological Measurement, 31,* 388–411.

Cherry, R. D., & Meyer, P. R. (1993). Reliability issues in holistic assessment. In M. M. Williamson & B. A. Huot (Eds.), *Validating holistic scoring for writing assessment: Theoretical and empirical foundations* (pp. 109–141). Cresskill, NJ: Hampton Press.

Chi, E. (2001). Comparing holistic and analytic scoring for performance assessment with many-facet Rasch model. *Journal of Applied Measurement, 2,* 379–388.

Chiu, C. W. T. (2001). *Scoring performance assessments based on judgements: Generalizability theory.* Boston, MA: Kluwer.

Chiu, C. W. T., & Wolfe, E. W. (2002). A method for analyzing sparse data matrices in the generalizability theory framework. *Applied Psychological Measurement, 26,* 321–338.

Chou, Y.-T., & Wang, W.-C. (2010). Checking dimensionality in item response models with principal component analysis on standardized residuals. *Educational and Psychological Measurement, 70,* 717–731.

Cizek, G. J. (2006). Standard setting. In S. M. Downing & T. M. Haladyna (Eds.), *Handbook of test development* (pp. 225–258). Mahwah, NJ: Erlbaum.

Cizek, G. J., & Bunch, M. B. (2007). *Standard setting: A guide to establishing and evaluating performance standards on tests.* Thousand Oaks, CA: Sage.

Clauser, B., & Linacre, J. M. (1999). Relating Cronbach and Rasch reliabilities. *Rasch Measurement Transactions, 13,* 696.

Cohen, J. (1960). A coefficient of agreement for nominal scales. *Educational and Psychological Measurement, 20,* 37–46.

Cohen, J. (1968). Weighted kappa: Nominal scale agreement with provision for scaled disagreement or partial credit. *Psychological Bulletin, 70,* 213–220.

Cohen, J., Chan, T., Jiang, T., & Seburn, M. (2008). Consistent estimation of Rasch item parameters and their standard errors under complex sample designs. *Applied Psychological Measurement, 32,* 289–310.

Cole, N. S. (1997). *The ETS gender study: How females and males perform in educational settings.* Princeton, NJ: Educational Testing Service.

Congdon, P. J., & McQueen, J. (2000a). The stability of rater severity in large-scale assessment programs. *Journal of Educational Measurement, 37,* 163–178.

Congdon, P. J., & McQueen, J. (2000b). Unmodeled rater discrimination error. In M. Wilson & G. Engelhard (Eds.), *Objective measurement: Theory into practice* (Vol. 5, pp. 165–180). Stamford, CT: Ablex.

Coniam, D. (2008). Problems affecting the use of raw scores: A comparison of raw scores and FACETS' fair average scores. In L. Taylor & C. J. Weir (Eds.), *Multilingualism and assessment: Achieving transparency, assuring quality, sustaining diversity – Proceedings of the ALTE Berlin Conference May 2005* (pp. 179–190). Cambridge, UK: Cambridge University Press.

Cooper, W. H. (1981). Ubiquitous halo. *Psychological Bulletin, 90,* 218–244.

Council of Europe. (2001). *Common European framework of reference for languages: Learning, teaching, assessment.* Cambridge, UK: Cambridge University Press.

Council of Europe. (2009). *Relating language examinations to the common European framework of reference for languages: Learning, teaching, assessment (CEFR): A manual.* Strasbourg, France: Council of Europe/Language Policy Division. Retrieved from http://www.coe.int/t/dg4/linguistic/manuel1_EN.asp?

Creswell, J. W., & Plano Clark, V. L. (2011). *Designing and conducting mixed methods research* (2nd ed.). Thousand Oaks, CA: Sage.

Crick, J. E., & Brennan, R. L. (2001). GENOVA: A general purpose analysis of variance system (Version 3.1) [Computer software]. Iowa City, IA: Iowa Testing Program.

Crisp, V. (2008). Exploring the nature of examiner thinking during the process of examination marking. *Cambridge Journal of Education, 38,* 247–264.

Cronbach, L. J., Gleser, G. C., Nanda, H., & Rajaratnam, N. (1972). *The dependability of behavioral measurements: Theory of generalizability for scores and profiles.* New York, NY: Wiley.

Cumming, A. (1990). Expertise in evaluating second language compositions. *Language Testing, 7,* 31–51.

Cumming, A., Kantor, R., & Powers, D. E. (2002). Decision making while rating ESL/EFL writing tasks: A descriptive framework. *Modern Language Journal, 86,* 67–96.

Curtis, D. D., & Boman, P. (2007). X-ray your data with Rasch. *International Education Journal, 8,* 249–259.

Davis, L. (2009). The influence of interlocutor proficiency in a paired oral assessment. *Language Testing, 26,* 367–396.

de Ayala, R. J. (2009). *The theory and practice of item response theory.* New York, NY: Guilford.

DeCarlo, L. T. (2005). A model of rater behavior in essay grading based on signal detection theory. *Journal of Educational Measurement, 42,* 53–76.

DeCarlo, L. T., Kim, Y. K., & Johnson, M. S. (2011). A hierarchical rater model for constructed responses, with a signal detection rater model. *Journal of Educational Measurement, 48,* 333–356.

de Gruijter, D. N. M., & van der Kamp, L. J. T. (2008). *Statistical test theory for the behavioral sciences.* Boca Raton, FL: Chapman & Hall/CRC.

de Jong, J., & Linacre, J. M. (1993). Estimation methods, statistical independence and global fit. *Rasch Measurement Transactions, 7*, 296–297.

DeMars, C. (2010). *Item response theory.* New York, NY: Oxford University Press.

Dewberry, C., Davies-Muir, A., & Newell, S. (2013). Impact and causes of rater severity/leniency in appraisals without postevaluation communication between raters and ratees. *International Journal of Selection and Assessment, 21*, 286–293.

Dobria, L. (2011). *Longitudinal rater modeling with splines* (Unpublished doctoral dissertation). University of Illinois at Chicago, Chicago, IL.

Dobria, L. (2012, April). *On the multilevel facets model for the analysis of rating data.* Paper presented at the Annual Meeting of the American Educational Research Association, Vancouver, Canada.

Doran, H., Bates, D., Bliese, P., & Dowling, M. (2007). Estimating the multilevel Rasch model: With the lme4 package. *Journal of Statistical Software, 20*(2).

Downing, S. M. (2005). Threats to the validity of clinical teaching assessments: What about rater error? *Medical Education, 39*, 350–355.

Downing, S. M., & Haladyna, T. M. (2004). Validity threats: Overcoming interference with proposed interpretations of assessment data. *Medical Education*, 38, 327–333.

Du, Y., & Brown, W. L. (2000). Raters and single prompt-to-prompt equating using the facets model in a writing performance assessment. In M. Wilson & G. Engelhard (Eds.), *Objective measurement: Theory into practice* (Vol. 5, pp. 97–111). Stamford, CT: Ablex.

Du, Y., & Wright, B. D. (1997). Effects of student characteristics in a large-scale direct writing assessment. In M. Wilson, G. Engelhard, & K. Draney (Eds.), *Objective measurement: Theory into practice* (Vol. 4, pp. 1–24). Stamford, CT: Ablex.

Du, Y., Wright, B. D., & Brown, W. L. (1996, April). *Differential facet functioning detection in direct writing assessment.* Paper presented at the Annual Meeting of the American Educational Research Association, New York, NY.

Eckes, T. (2004). Beurteilerübereinstimmung und Beurteilerstrenge: Eine Multifacetten-Rasch-Analyse von Leistungsbeurteilungen im „Test Deutsch als Fremdsprache“ (TestDaF) [Rater agreement and rater severity: A many-facet Rasch analysis of performance assessments in the „Test of German as a Foreign Language (TestDaF)“]. *Diagnostica, 50*, 65–77.

Eckes, T. (2005a). Evaluation von Beurteilungen: Psychometrische Qualitätssicherung mit dem Multifacetten-Rasch-Modell [Evaluation of ratings: Psychometric quality assurance via many-facet Rasch measurement]. *Zeitschrift für Psychologie, 213*, 77–96.

Eckes, T. (2005b). Examining rater effects in TestDaF writing and speaking performance assessments: A many-facet Rasch analysis. *Language Assessment Quarterly, 2*, 197–221.

Eckes, T. (2008a). Assuring the quality of TestDaF examinations: A psychometric modeling approach. In L. Taylor & C. J. Weir (Eds.), *Multilingualism and assessment: Achieving transparency, assuring quality, sustaining diversity – Proceedings of the ALTE Berlin Conference May 2005* (pp. 157–178). Cambridge, UK: Cambridge University Press.

Eckes, T. (2008b). Rater types in writing performance assessments: A classification approach to rater variability. *Language Testing, 25*, 155–185.

Eckes, T. (2009a). Many-facet Rasch measurement. In S. Takala (Ed.), *Reference supplement to the manual for relating language examinations to the Common European Framework of Reference for Languages: Learning, teaching, assessment* (Section H). Strasbourg, France: Council of Europe/Language Policy Division. Retrieved from http://www.coe.int/t/dg4/linguistic/manuel1_EN.asp?#Reference

Eckes, T. (2009b). On common ground? How raters perceive scoring criteria in oral proficiency testing. In A. Brown & K. Hill (Eds.), *Tasks and criteria in performance assessment: Proceedings of the 28th Language Testing Research Colloquium* (pp. 43–73). Frankfurt, Germany: Lang.

Eckes, T. (2010a). Die Beurteilung sprachlicher Kompetenz auf dem Prüfstand: Fairness in der beurteilergestützten Leistungsmessung [Putting ratings of language competence to the test: Fairness in rater-mediated performance assessment]. In K. Aguado, K. Schramm, & H. J. Vollmer (Eds.), *Fremdsprachliches Handeln beobachten, messen und evaluieren* (pp. 65–97). Frankfurt, Germany: Lang.

Eckes, T. (2010b). The TestDaF implementation of the SOPI: Design, analysis, and evaluation of a semi-direct speaking test. In L. Araújo (Ed.), *Computer-based assessment (CBA) of foreign language speaking skills* (pp. 63–83). Luxembourg: Publications Office of the European Union.

Eckes, T. (2012). Operational rater types in writing assessment: Linking rater cognition to rater behavior. *Language Assessment Quarterly, 9*, 270–292.

Elbow, P., & Yancey, K. B. (1994). On the nature of holistic scoring: An inquiry composed on email. *Assessing Writing, 1*, 91–107.

Elder, C., Barkhuizen, G., Knoch, U., & von Randow, J. (2007). Evaluating rater responses to an online training program for L2 writing assessment. *Language Testing, 24*, 37–64.

Elder, C., Knoch, U., Barkhuizen, G., & von Randow, J. (2005). Individual feedback to enhance rater training: Does it work? *Language Assessment Quarterly, 2,* 175–196.

Embretson, S. E., & Reise, S. P. (2000). *Item response theory for psychologists.* Mahwah, NJ: Erlbaum.

Emerling, F. (1991). Identifying ethnicity and gender from anonymous essays. *Community College Review, 19,* 29–33.

Engelhard, G. (1992). The measurement of writing ability with a many-faceted Rasch model. *Applied Measurement in Education, 5,* 171–191.

Engelhard, G. (1994). Examining rater errors in the assessment of written composition with a many-faceted Rasch model. *Journal of Educational Measurement, 31,* 93–112.

Engelhard, G. (1997). Constructing rater and task banks for performance assessments. *Journal of Outcome Measurement, 1,* 19–33.

Engelhard, G. (2002). Monitoring raters in performance assessments. In G. Tindal & T. M. Haladyna (Eds.), *Large-scale assessment programs for all students: Validity, technical adequacy, and implementation* (pp. 261–287). Mahwah, NJ: Erlbaum.

Engelhard, G. (2007a). Differential rater functioning. *Rasch Measurement Transactions, 21,* 1124.

Engelhard, G. (2007b). Evaluating bookmark judgments. *Rasch Measurement Transactions, 21,* 1097–1098.

Engelhard, G. (2008a). Historical perspectives on invariant measurement: Guttman, Rasch, and Mokken. *Measurement: Interdisciplinary Research and Perspective, 6,* 155–189.

Engelhard, G. (2008b). Standard errors for performance standards based on bookmark judgments. *Rasch Measurement Transactions, 21,* 1132–1133.

Engelhard, G. (2011). Evaluating the bookmark judgments of standard-setting panelists. *Educational and Psychological Measurement, 71,* 909–924.

Engelhard, G. (2013). *Invariant measurement: Using Rasch models in the social, behavioral, and health sciences.* New York, NY: Routledge.

Engelhard, G., & Anderson, D. W. (1998). A binomial trials model for examining the ratings of standard-setting judges. *Applied Measurement in Education, 11,* 209–230.

Engelhard, G., & Cramer, S. E. (1997). Using Rasch measurement to evaluate the ratings of standard-setting judges. In M. Wilson, G. Engelhard, & K. Draney (Eds.), *Objective measurement: Theory into practice* (Vol. 4, pp. 97–112). Greenwich, CT: Ablex.

Engelhard, G., & Gordon, B. (2000). Setting and evaluating performance standards for high stakes writing assessments. In M. Wilson & G. Engelhard (Eds.), *Objective measurement: Theory into practice* (Vol. 5, pp. 3–14). Stamford, CT: Ablex.

Engelhard, G., Gordon, B., & Gabrielson, S. (1991). The influences of mode of discourse, experiential demand, and gender on the quality of student writing. *Research in the Teaching of English, 26*, 315–336.

Engelhard, G., & Myford, C. M. (2003). *Monitoring faculty consultant performance in the Advanced Placement English Literature and Composition Program with a many-faceted Rasch model* (College Board Research Report No. 2003–1). New York, NY: College Entrance Examination Board.

Engelhard, G., & Stone, G. E. (1998). Evaluating the quality of ratings obtained from standard-setting judges. *Educational and Psychological Measurement, 58*, 179–196.

Eva, K. W., Rosenfeld, J., Reiter, H. I., & Norman, G. R. (2004). An admissions OSCE: The multiple mini-interview. *Medical Education, 38*, 314–326.

Ferne, T., & Rupp, A. (2007). A synthesis of 15 years of research on DIF in language testing: Methodological advances, challenges, and recommendations. *Language Assessment Quarterly, 4*, 113–148.

Fischer, G. H. (1973). The linear logistic test model as an instrument in educational research. *Acta Psychologica, 37*, 359–374.

Fischer, G. H. (1995a). Derivations of the Rasch model. In G. H. Fischer & I. W. Molenaar (Eds.), *Rasch models: Foundations, recent developments, and applications* (pp. 15–38). New York, NY: Springer.

Fischer, G. H. (1995b). The linear logistic test model. In G. H. Fischer & I. W. Molenaar (Eds.), *Rasch models: Foundations, recent developments, and applications* (pp. 131–155). New York, NY: Springer.

Fischer, G. H. (2005). Linear logistic test models. *Encyclopedia of Social Measurement, 2*, 505–514.

Fischer, G. H. (2007). Rasch models. In C. R. Rao & S. Sinharay (Eds.), *Psychometrics* (*Handbook of statistics*, Vol. 26, pp. 515–585). Amsterdam, The Netherlands: Elsevier.

Fischer, G. H. (2010). The Rasch model in Europe: A history. *Rasch Measurement Transactions, 24*, 1294–1295.

Fischer, G. H., & Ponocny-Seliger, E. (2003). Structural Rasch modeling: Handbook of the usage of LPCM-WIN (Version 1.0) [Computer software]. Groningen, The Netherlands: Science Plus Group.

Fischer, G. H., & Scheiblechner, H. H. (1970). Algorithmen und Programme für das probabilistische Testmodell von Rasch [Algorithms and programs for Rasch's probabilistic test model]. *Psychologische Beiträge, 12,* 23–51.

Fisher, W. P. (1993). Robustness and invariance. *Rasch Measurement Transactions, 7,* 295.

Fisicaro, S. A., & Lance, C. E. (1990). Implications of three causal models for the measurement of halo error. *Applied Psychological Measurement, 14,* 419–429.

Fleiss, J. L., Levin, B., & Paik, M. C. (2003). *Statistical methods for rates and proportions* (3rd ed.). Hoboken, NJ: Wiley.

Freedman, S. W., & Calfee, R. C. (1983). Holistic assessment of writing: Experimental design and cognitive theory. In P. Mosenthal, L. Tamor, & S. A. Walmsley (Eds.), *Research on writing: Principles and methods* (pp. 75–98). New York, NY: Longman.

Fulcher, G. (2003). *Testing second language speaking.* London: Pearson Education.

Galaczi, E. D. (2010). Face-to-face and computer-based assessment of speaking: Challenges and opportunities. In L. Araújo (Ed.), *Computer-based assessment (CBA) of foreign language speaking skills* (pp. 29–51). Luxembourg: Publications Office of the European Union.

Gamaroff, R. (2000). Rater reliability in language assessment: The bug of all bears. *System, 28,* 31–53.

Govaerts, M. J. B., Van de Wiel, M. W. J., Schuwirth, L. W. T., Van der Vleuten, C. P. M., & Muijtjens, A. M. M. (2013). Workplace-based assessment: Raters' performance theories and constructs. *Advances in Health Sciences Education, 18,* 375–396.

Guilford, J. P. (1936). *Psychometric methods.* New York, NY: McGraw-Hill.

Guo, S. (2014). Correction of rater effects in longitudinal research with a cross-classified random effects model. *Applied Psychological Measurement, 38,* 37–60.

Gyagenda, I. S., & Engelhard, G. (2009). Using classical and modern measurement theories to explore rater, domain, and gender influences on student writing ability. *Journal of Applied Measurement, 10,* 225–246.

Haertel, E. H. (2006). Reliability. In R. L. Brennan (Ed.), *Educational measurement* (4th ed., pp. 65–110). Westport, CT: American Council on Education/Praeger.

Haladyna, T. M., & Downing, S. M. (2004). Construct-irrelevant variance in high-stakes testing. *Educational Measurement: Issues and Practice, 23,* 17–27.

Hambleton, R. K., & Pitoniak, M. J. (2006). Setting performance standards. In R. L. Brennan (Ed.), *Educational measurement* (4th ed., pp. 433–470). Westport, CT: American Council on Education/Praeger.

Hamp-Lyons, L. (2007). Worrying about rating. *Assessing Writing, 12*, 1–9.

Harasym, P. H., Woloschuk, W., & Cunning, L. (2008). Undesired variance due to examiner stringency/leniency effect in communication skill scores assessed in OSCEs. *Advances in Health Sciences Education, 13*, 617–632.

Hartig, J., & Höhler, J. (2008). Representation of competencies in multidimensional IRT models with within-item and between-item multidimensionality. *Zeitschrift für Psychologie/Journal of Psychology, 216*, 89–101.

Haswell, R. H., & Haswell, J. T. (1996). Gender bias and critique of student writing. *Assessing Writing, 3*, 31–83.

Hayes, A. F., & Krippendorff, K. (2007). Answering the call for a standard reliability measure for coding data. *Communication Methods and Measures, 1*, 77–89.

Hays, W. L. (1994). *Statistics* (5th ed.). Belmont, CA: Wadsworth.

He, T.-H., Gou, W. J., Chien, Y.-C., Chen, I-S. J., & Chang, S.-M. (2013). Multi-faceted Rasch measurement and bias patterns in EFL writing performance assessment. *Psychological Reports: Measures & Statistics, 112*, 469–485.

Hedges, L. V., & Nowell, A. (1995). Sex differences in mental test scores, variability and number of high-scoring individuals. *Science, 269*, 41–45.

Hedges, L. V., & Olkin, I. (1985). *Statistical methods for meta-analysis*. San Diego, CA: Academic Press.

Henning, G. (1989). Meanings and implications of the principle of local independence. *Language Testing, 6*, 95–108.

Henning, G. (1992). Dimensionality and construct validity of language tests. *Language Testing, 9*, 1–11.

Henning, G. (1996). Accounting for nonsystematic error in performance ratings. *Language Testing, 13*, 53–61.

Hombo, C. M., Donoghue, J. R., & Thayer, D. T. (2001). *A simulation study of the effect of rater designs on ability estimation* (Research Report, RR-01-05). Princeton, NJ: Educational Testing Service.

Hooker, G., Finkelman, M., & Schwartzman, A. (2009). Paradoxical results in multidimensional item response theory. *Psychometrika, 74*, 419–442.

Hoskens, M., & Wilson, M. (2001). Real-time feedback on rater drift in constructed-response items: An example from the Golden State Examination. *Journal of Educational Measurement, 38*, 121–145.

Houston, J. E., & Myford, C. M. (2009). Judges' perception of candidates' organization and communication, in relation to oral certification examination ratings. *Academic Medicine, 84*, 1603–1609.

Houston, W. M., Raymond, M. R., & Svec, J. C. (1991). Adjustments for rater effects in performance assessment. *Applied Psychological Measurement, 15*, 409–421.

Hoyt, W. T. (2000). Rater bias in psychological research: When is it a problem and what can we do about it? *Psychological Methods, 5*, 64–86.

Hoyt, W. T., & Kerns, M.-D. (1999). Magnitude and moderators of bias in observer ratings: A meta-analysis. *Psychological Methods, 4*, 403–424.

Hsieh, M. (2013). An application of multifaceted Rasch measurement in the Yes/No Angoff standard setting procedure. *Language Testing, 30*, 491–512.

Hung, L.-F., & Wang, W.-C. (2012). The generalized multilevel facets model for longitudinal data. *Journal of Educational and Behavioral Statistics, 37*, 231–255.

Hyde, J. S., & Linn, M. C. (1988). Gender differences in verbal ability: A meta-analysis. *Psychological Bulletin, 104*, 53–69.

Iramaneerat, C., Smith, E. V., & Smith, R. M. (2008). An introduction to Rasch measurement. In J. W. Osborne (Ed.), *Best practices in quantitative methods* (pp. 50–70). Los Angeles, CA: Sage.

Iramaneerat, C., & Yudkowsky, R. (2007). Rater errors in a clinical skills assessment of medical students. *Evaluation and the Health Professions, 30*, 266–283.

Iramaneerat, C., Yudkowsky, R., Myford, C. M., & Downing, S. M. (2008). Quality control of an OSCE using generalizability theory and many-faceted Rasch measurement. *Advances in Health Sciences Education, 13*, 479–493.

James, L. R., Demaree, R. G., & Wolf, G. (1984). Estimating within-group interrater reliability with and without response bias. *Journal of Applied Psychology, 69*, 85–98.

James, L. R., Demaree, R. G., & Wolf, G. (1993). r_{wg}: An assessment of within-group interrater agreement. *Journal of Applied Psychology, 78*, 306–309.

Jiao, H., Wang, S., & Kamata, A. (2007). Modeling local item dependence with the hierarchical generalized linear model. In E. V. Smith & R. M. Smith (Eds.), *Rasch measurement: Advanced and specialized applications* (pp. 390–404). Maple Grove, MN: JAM Press.

Johnson, R. L., Penny, J. A., & Gordon, B. (2009). *Assessing performance: Designing, scoring, and validating performance tasks.* New York, NY: Guilford.

Johnson, R. L., Penny, J. A., Gordon, B., Shumate, S. R., & Fisher, S. P. (2005). Resolving score differences in the rating of writing samples: Does discussion improve the accuracy of scores? *Language Assessment Quarterly, 2*, 117–146.

Kaftandjieva, F. (2004). Standard setting. In S. Takala (Ed.), *Reference supplement to the preliminary pilot version of the manual for relating language examinations to the Common European Framework of Reference for Languages: Learning, teaching, assessment* (Section B). Strasbourg, France: Council of Europe/ Language Policy Division. Retrieved from http://www.coe.int/t/dg4/linguistic/manuel1_EN.asp?#Reference

Kaftandjieva, F. (2010). *Methods for setting cut scores in criterion-referenced achievement tests: A comparative analysis of six recent methods with an application to tests of reading in EFL.* Arnhem, The Netherlands: EALTA.

Kaliski, P. K., Wind, S. A., Engelhard, G., Morgan, D. L., Plake, B. S., & Reshetar, R. A. (2013). Using the many-faceted Rasch model to evaluate standard setting judgments: An illustration with the Advanced Placement Environmental Science exam. *Educational and Psychological Measurement, 73,* 386–411.

Kamata, A., & Cheong, Y. F. (2007). Multilevel Rasch models. In M. von Davier & C. H. Carstensen (Eds.), *Multivariate and mixture distribution Rasch models: Extensions and applications* (pp. 217–232). New York, NY: Springer.

Kane, M. T. (1992). An argument-based approach to validation. *Psychological Bulletin, 112,* 527–535.

Kane, M. (1994). Validating the performance standards associated with passing scores. *Review of Educational Research, 64,* 425–461.

Kane, M. T. (2001). So much remains the same: Conception and status of validation in setting standards. In G. J. Cizek (Ed.), *Setting performance standards: Concepts, methods, and perspectives* (pp. 53–88). Mahwah, NJ: Erlbaum.

Kane, M. T. (2006). Validation. In R. L. Brennan (Ed.), *Educational measurement* (4th ed., pp. 17–64). Westport, CT: American Council on Education/Praeger.

Kane, M. T. (2013). Validating the interpretations and uses of test scores. *Journal of Educational Measurement, 50,* 1–73.

Karabatsos, G. (2000). A critique of Rasch residual fit statistics. *Journal of Applied Measurement, 1,* 152–176.

Karabatsos, G. (2003). Comparing the aberrant response detection performance of thirty-six person-fit statistics. *Applied Measurement in Education, 16,* 277–298.

Kecker, G., & Eckes, T. (2010). Putting the Manual to the test: The TestDaF–CEFR linking project. In W. Martyniuk (Ed.), *Aligning tests with the CEFR: Reflections on using the Council of Europe's draft Manual* (pp. 50–79). Cambridge, UK: Cambridge University Press.

Kempf, W. F. (1972). Probabilistische Modelle experimentalpsychologischer Versuchssituationen [Probabilistic models of designs in experimental psychology]. *Psychologische Beiträge, 14,* 16–37.

Kiefer, T., Robitzsch, A., & Wu, M. (2014). Package ‚TAM' (Version 1.0–3) [Computer software and manual]. Retrieved from http://cran.R-project.org/web/packages/TAM/index.html

Kim, S. C., & Wilson, M. (2009). A comparative analysis of the ratings in performance assessment using generalizability theory and the many-facet Rasch model. *Journal of Applied Measurement, 10,* 408–423.

Kim, Y.-H. (2009). An investigation into native and non-native teachers' judgments of oral English performance: A mixed methods approach. *Language Testing, 26*, 187–217.

Kingsbury, F. A. (1922). Analyzing ratings and training raters. *Journal of Personnel Research, 1*, 377–383.

Kline, T. L., Schmidt, K. M., & Bowles, R. (2006). Using LinLog and FACETS to model item components in the LLTM. *Journal of Applied Measurement, 7*, 74–91.

Knoch, U. (2009a). Diagnostic assessment of writing: A comparison of two rating scales. *Language Testing, 26*, 275–304.

Knoch, U. (2009b). *Diagnostic writing assessment: The development and validation of a rating scale*. Frankfurt, Germany: Lang.

Knoch, U. (2011). Investigating the effectiveness of individualized feedback to rating behavior: A longitudinal study. *Language Testing, 28*, 179–200.

Knoch, U., Read, J., & von Randow, J. (2007). Re-training writing raters online: How does it compare with face-to-face training? *Assessing Writing, 12*, 26–43.

Kolen, M. J. (2007). Data collection designs and linking procedures. In N. J. Dorans, M. Pommerich, & P. W. Holland (Eds.), *Linking and aligning scores and scales* (pp. 31–55). New York, NY: Springer.

Kolen, M. J., & Brennan, R. L. (2004). *Test equating, scaling, and linking: Methods and practices* (2nd ed.). New York, NY: Springer.

Kondo-Brown, K. (2002). A FACETS analysis of rater bias in measuring Japanese second language writing performance. *Language Testing, 19*, 3–31.

Koskey, K. L. K., & Stewart, V. C. (2014). A concurrent mixed methods approach to examining the quantitative and qualitative meaningfulness of absolute magnitude estimation scales in survey research. *Journal of Mixed Methods Research, 8*, 180–202.

Kozaki, Y. (2004). Using GENOVA and FACETS to set multiple standards on performance assessment for certification in medical translation from Japanese into English. *Language Testing, 21*, 1–27.

Kozaki, Y. (2010). An alternative decision-making procedure for performance assessments: Using the multifaceted Rasch model to generate cut estimates. *Language Assessment Quarterly, 7*, 75–95.

Kubinger, K. D. (2005). Psychological test calibration using the Rasch model: Some critical suggestions on traditional approaches. *International Journal of Testing, 5*, 377–394.

Kubinger, K. D. (2009). Applications of the linear logistic test model in psychometric research. *Educational and Psychological Measurement, 69*, 232–244.

Lai, E. R., Wolfe, E. W., & Vickers, D. (2015). Differentiation of illusory and true halo in writing scores. *Educational and Psychological Measurement, 75*, 102–125.

Lamprianou, I. (2006). The stability of marker characteristics across tests of the same subject and across subjects. *Journal of Applied Measurement, 7*, 192–205.

Lamprianou, I. (2008). High stakes tests with self-selected essay questions: Addressing issues of fairness. *International Journal of Testing, 8*, 55–89.

Lamprianou, I. (2013). Application of single-level and multi-level Rasch models using the lme4 package. *Journal of Applied Measurement, 14*, 79–90.

Landy, F. J., & Farr, J. L. (1980). Performance rating. *Psychological Bulletin, 87*, 72–107.

Lane, S., & Stone, C. A. (2006). Performance assessment. In R. L. Brennan (Ed.), *Educational measurement* (4th ed., pp. 387–431). Westport, CT: American Council on Education/Praeger.

Lazaraton, A. (2008). Utilizing qualitative methods for assessment. In E. Shohamy & N. H. Hornberger (Eds.), *Encyclopedia of language and education: Vol. 7. Language testing and assessment* (2nd ed., pp. 197–209). New York, NY: Springer.

LeBreton, J. M., & Senter, J. L. (2008). Answers to 20 questions about interrater reliability and interrater agreement. *Organizational Research Methods, 11*, 815–852.

Leckie, G., & Baird, J.-A. (2011). Rater effects on essay scoring: A multilevel analysis of severity drift, central tendency, and rater experience. *Journal of Educational Measurement, 48*, 399–418.

Lewin, K. (1951). *Field theory in social science: Selected theoretical papers* (D. Cartwright, Ed.). New York, NY: Harper & Row.

Lewis, D. M., Mitzel, H. C., Mercado, R. L., & Schulz, E. M. (2012). The Bookmark standard setting procedure. In G. J. Cizek (Ed.), *Setting performance standards: Foundations, methods, and innovations* (2nd ed., pp. 225–253). New York, NY: Routledge.

Lim, G. S. (2011). The development and maintenance of rating quality in performance writing assessment: A longitudinal study of new and experienced raters. *Language Testing, 28*, 543–560.

Linacre, J. M. (1989). *Many-facet Rasch measurement.* Chicago: MESA Press.

Linacre, J. M. (1994). Sample size and item calibration [or person measure] stability. *Rasch Measurement Transactions, 7*, 328.

Linacre, J. M. (1996a). Generalizability theory and many-facet Rasch measurement. In G. Engelhard & M. Wilson (Eds.), *Objective measurement: Theory into practice* (Vol. 3, pp. 85–98). Norwood, NJ: Ablex.

Linacre, J. M. (1996b). True-score reliability or Rasch validity? *Rasch Measurement Transactions, 9,* 455.

Linacre, J. M. (1997a). Investigating judge local independence. *Rasch Measurement Transactions, 11,* 546–547.

Linacre, J. M. (1997b). Is Rasch general enough? *Rasch Measurement Transactions, 11,* 555.

Linacre, J. M. (1997c). KR-20/Cronbach Alpha or Rasch reliability: Which tells the "truth"? *Rasch Measurement Transactions, 11,* 580–581.

Linacre, J. M. (1998a). Rating, judges and fairness. *Rasch Measurement Transactions, 12,* 630–631.

Linacre, J. M. (1998b). Structure in Rasch residuals: Why principal components analysis (PCA)? *Rasch Measurement Transactions, 12,* 636.

Linacre, J. M. (1999). Investigating rating scale category utility. *Journal of Outcome Measurement, 3,* 103–122.

Linacre, J. M. (2001). Generalizability theory and Rasch measurement. *Rasch Measurement Transactions, 15,* 806–807.

Linacre, J. M. (2002a). Facets, factors, elements and levels. *Rasch Measurement Transactions, 16,* 880.

Linacre, J. M. (2002b). Judge ratings with forced agreement. *Rasch Measurement Transactions, 16,* 857–858.

Linacre, J. M. (2002c). What do infit and outfit, mean-square and standardized mean? *Rasch Measurement Transactions, 16,* 878.

Linacre, J. M. (2003a). The hierarchical rater model from a Rasch perspective. *Rasch Measurement Transactions, 17,* 928.

Linacre, J. M. (2003b). Size vs. significance: Infit and outfit mean-square and standardized chi-square fit statistic. *Rasch Measurement Transactions, 17,* 918.

Linacre, J. M. (2004a). Estimation methods for Rasch measures. In E. V. Smith & R. M. Smith (Eds.), *Introduction to Rasch measurement* (pp. 25–47). Maple Grove, MN: JAM Press.

Linacre, J. M. (2004b). Optimizing rating scale category effectiveness. In E. V. Smith & R. M. Smith (Eds.), *Introduction to Rasch measurement* (pp. 258–278). Maple Grove, MN: JAM Press.

Linacre, J. M. (2004c). Rasch model estimation: Further topics. In E. V. Smith & R. M. Smith (Eds.), *Introduction to Rasch measurement* (pp. 48–72). Maple Grove, MN: JAM Press.

Linacre, J. M. (2005). Standard errors: Means, measures, origins and anchor values. *Rasch Measurement Transactions, 19,* 1030.

Linacre, J. M. (2006a). Demarcating category intervals. *Rasch Measurement Transactions, 19,* 1041–1043.

Linacre, J. M. (2006b). Item discrimination and Rasch-Andrich thresholds. *Rasch Measurement Transactions, 20,* 1054.

Linacre, J. M. (2009). *A user's guide to FACFORM: Data formatter for FACETS Rasch-model computer programs.* Chicago: Winsteps.com. Retrieved from http://www.winsteps.com/facets.htm

Linacre, J. M. (2010a). Removing Rasch misfit and cleaning windows. *Rasch Measurement Transactions, 23,* 1241.

Linacre, J. M. (2010b). Transitional categories and usefully disordered thresholds. *Online Educational Research Journal, 1*(3).

Linacre, J. M. (2011, June). *Constructing valid performance assessments: The view from the shoulders of the giants.* Samuel J. Messick Memorial Lecture presented at the 33rd Language Testing Research Colloquium, Michigan, MI. Retrieved from http://www.rasch.org/memo85.pdf

Linacre, J. M. (2012). *Many-facet Rasch measurement: Facets tutorial 2 – Fit analysis and measurement models.* Retrieved from http://www.winsteps.com/tutorials.htm

Linacre, J. M. (2014a). Facets Rasch measurement computer program (Version 3.71.4) [Computer software]. Chicago: Winsteps.com.

Linacre, J. M. (2014b). *A user's guide to FACETS: Rasch-model computer programs.* Chicago: Winsteps.com. Retrieved from http://www.winsteps.com/facets.htm

Linacre, J. M. (2014c). *A user's guide to WINSTEPS: Rasch-model computer programs.* Chicago: Winsteps.com. Retrieved from http://www.winsteps.com/winsteps.htm

Linacre, J. M., Engelhard, G., Tatum, D. S., & Myford, C. M. (1994). Measurement with judges: Many-faceted conjoint measurement. *International Journal of Educational Research, 21,* 569–577.

Linacre, J. M., & Wright, B. D. (1989). The length of a logit. *Rasch Measurement Transactions, 3,* 54–55.

Linacre, J. M., & Wright, B. D. (2002). Construction of measures from many-facet data. *Journal of Applied Measurement, 3,* 484–509.

Lissitz, R. W. (Ed.). (2009). *The concept of validity: Revisions, new directions, and applications.* Charlotte, NC: Information Age.

Liu, O. L., Wilson, M., & Paek, I. (2008). A multidimensional Rasch analysis of gender differences in PISA mathematics. *Journal of Applied Measurement, 9*, 18–35.

Loevinger, J. (1954). The attenuation paradox in test theory. *Psychological Bulletin, 51*, 493–504.

Longford, N. T. (1996). Reconciling experts' differences in setting cut scores for pass-fail decisions. *Journal of Educational and Behavioral Statistics, 21*, 203–213.

Looney, M. A. (2012). Judging anomalies at the 2010 Olympics in men's figure skating. *Measurement in Physical Education and Exercise Science, 16*, 55–68.

López-Pina, J. A., & Hidalgo-Montesinos, M. D. (2005). Fitting Rasch model using appropriateness measure statistics. *Spanish Journal of Psychology, 8*, 100–110.

Lord, F. M., & Novick, M. R. (1968). *Statistical theories of mental test scores*. Reading, MA: Addison-Wesley.

Ludlow, L. H., & Haley, S. M. (1995). Rasch model logits: Interpretation, use, and transformation. *Educational and Psychological Measurement, 55*, 967–975.

Lumley, T. (2005). *Assessing second language writing: The rater's perspective.* Frankfurt, Germany: Lang.

Lumley, T., & Brown, A. (2005). Research methods in language testing. In E. Hinkel (Ed.), *Handbook of research in second language teaching and learning* (pp. 833–855). Mahwah, NJ: Erlbaum.

Lumley, T., Lynch, B. K., & McNamara, T. F. (1994). A new approach to standard-setting in language assessment. *Melbourne Papers in Language Testing, 3*, 19–39.

Lumley, T., & McNamara, T. F. (1995). Rater characteristics and rater bias: Implications for training. *Language Testing, 12*, 54–71.

Lunz, M. E. (2000). Setting standards on performance examinations. In M. Wilson & G. Engelhard (Eds.), *Objective measurement: Theory into practice* (Vol. 5, pp. 181–199). Stamford, CT: Ablex.

Lunz, M. E., & Linacre, J. M. (1998). Measurement designs using multifacet Rasch modeling. In G. A. Marcoulides (Ed.), *Modern methods for business research* (pp. 47–77). Mahwah, NJ: Erlbaum.

Lunz, M. E., & Schumacker, R. E. (1997). Scoring and analysis of performance examinations: A comparison of methods and interpretations. *Journal of Outcome Measurement, 1*, 219–238.

Lunz, M. E., Stahl, J. A., & Wright, B. D. (1996). The invariance of judge severity calibrations. In G. Engelhard & M. Wilson (Eds.), *Objective measurement: Theory into practice* (Vol. 3, pp. 99–112). Norwood, NJ: Ablex.

Lunz, M. E., & Suanthong, S. (2011). Equating of multi-facet tests across administrations. *Journal of Applied Measurement, 12*, 124–134.

Lunz, M. E., Wright, B. D., & Linacre, J. M. (1990). Measuring the impact of judge severity on examination scores. *Applied Measurement in Education, 3*, 331–345.

Luo, G. (2005). The relationship between the rating scale and partial credit models and the implication of disordered thresholds of the Rasch models for polytomous responses. *Journal of Applied Measurement, 6*, 443–455.

Lynch, B. K., & McNamara, T. F. (1998). Using G-theory and many-facet Rasch measurement in the development of performance assessments of the ESL speaking skills of immigrants. *Language Testing, 15*, 158–180.

MacMillan, P. D. (2000). Classical, generalizability, and multifaceted Rasch detection of interrater variability in large, sparse data sets. *Journal of Experimental Education, 68*, 167–190.

Mair, P., & Hatzinger, R. (2007a). CML based estimation of extended Rasch models with the eRm package in R. *Psychology Science, 49*, 26–43.

Mair, P., & Hatzinger, R. (2007b). Extended Rasch modeling: The eRm package for the application of IRT models in R. *Journal of Statistical Software, 20*(9).

Mair, P., Hatzinger, R., & Maier, M. J. (2014). Package 'eRm' (Version 0.15–4) [Computer software and manual]. Retrieved from http://cran.R-project.org/web/packages/eRm/index.html

Marcoulides, G. A. (2000). Generalizability theory. In H. E. A. Tinsley & S. D. Brown (Eds.), *Handbook of applied multivariate statistics and mathematical modeling* (pp. 527–551). San Diego, CA: Academic Press.

Mariano, L. T., & Junker, B. W. (2007). Covariates of the rating process in hierarchical models for multiple ratings of test items. *Journal of Educational and Behavioral Statistics, 32*, 287–314.

Markus, K. A., & Borsboom, D. (2013). *Frontiers of test validity theory: Measurement, causation, and meaning.* New York, NY: Routledge.

Masters, G. N. (1982). A Rasch model for partial credit scoring. *Psychometrika, 47*, 149–174.

Masters, G. N. (2010). The partial credit model. In M. L. Nering & R. Ostini (Eds.), *Handbook of polytomous item response theory models* (pp. 109–122). New York, NY: Routledge.

Mattern, K., Camara, W., & Kobrin, J. L. (2007). *SAT writing: An overview of research and psychometrics to date* (RN-32). New York, NY: College Board.

McGraw, K. O., & Wong, S. P. (1996). Forming inferences about some intraclass correlation coefficients. *Psychological Methods, 1*, 30–46.

McManus, I. C., Thompson, M., & Mollon, J. (2006). Assessment of examiner leniency and stringency ('hawk-dove effect') in the MRCP(UK) clinical examination (PACES) using multi-facet Rasch modelling. *BMC Medical Education, 6*(42).

McNamara, T. F. (1995). Modelling performance: Opening Pandora's box. *Applied Linguistics, 16,* 159–179.

McNamara, T. F. (1996). *Measuring second language performance.* London: Longman.

McNamara, T. F. (2000). *Language testing.* Oxford, UK: Oxford University Press.

McNamara, T. F. (2011). Applied linguistics and measurement: A dialogue. *Language Testing, 28,* 435–440.

McNamara, T. (2014). 30 years on—Evolution or revolution? *Language Assessment Quarterly, 11,* 226–232.

McNamara, T., & Knoch, U. (2012). The Rasch wars: The emergence of Rasch measurement in language testing. *Language Testing, 29,* 555–576.

McNamara, T. F., & Roever, C. (2006). *Language testing: The social dimension.* Malden, MA: Blackwell.

Meijer, R. R., & Sijtsma, K. (2001). Methodology review: Evaluating person fit. *Applied Psychological Measurement, 25,* 107–135.

Messick, S. (1989). Validity. In R. L. Linn (Ed.), *Educational measurement* (3rd ed., pp. 13–103). New York, NY: Macmillan.

Messick, S. (1995). Validity of psychological assessment: Validation of inferences from persons' responses and performances as scientific inquiry into score meaning. *American Psychologist, 50,* 741–749.

Micko, H. C. (1969). A psychological scale for reaction time measurement. *Acta Psychologica, 30,* 324–335.

Micko, H. C. (1970). Eine Verallgemeinerung des Meßmodells von Rasch mit einer Anwendung auf die Psychophysik der Reaktionen [A generalization of Rasch's measurement model with an application to the psychophysics of reactions]. *Psychologische Beiträge, 12,* 4–22.

Mitzel, H. C., Lewis, D. M., Patz, R. J., & Green, D. R. (2001). The bookmark procedure: Psychological perspectives. In G. J. Cizek (Ed.), *Setting performance standards: Concepts, methods, and perspectives* (pp. 249–281). Mahwah, NJ: Erlbaum.

Molenaar, I. W. (1995). Estimation of item parameters. In G. H. Fischer & I. W. Molenaar (Eds.), *Rasch models: Foundations, recent developments, and applications* (pp. 39–51). New York, NY: Springer.

Morrow, K. (1979). Communicative language testing: Revolution or evolution? In C. J. Brumfit & K. Johnson (Eds.), *The communicative approach to language teaching* (pp. 143–157). Oxford, UK: Oxford University Press.

Morgan, G. B., Zhu, M., Johnson, R. L., & Hodge, K. J. (2014). Interrater reliability estimators commonly used in scoring language assessments: A Monte Carlo investigation of estimator accuracy. *Language Assessment Quarterly, 11*, 304–324.

Muckle, T. J., & Karabatsos, G. (2009). Hierarchical generalized linear models for the analysis of judge ratings. *Journal of Educational Measurement, 46*, 198–219.

Mulqueen, C., Baker, D. P., & Dismukes, R. K. (2002). Pilot instructor rater training: The utility of the multifacet item response theory model. *International Journal of Aviation Psychology, 12*, 287–303.

Mun, E. Y. (2005). Rater agreement – weighted kappa. In B. S. Everitt & D. Howell (Eds.), *Encyclopedia of statistics in behavioral science* (Vol. 3, pp. 1714–1715). New York, NY: Wiley.

Muraki, E. (1992). A generalized partial credit model: Application of an EM algorithm. *Applied Psychological Measurement, 16*, 159–176.

Murphy, K. R., & Cleveland, J. N. (1995). *Understanding performance appraisal: Social, organizational, and goal-based perspectives.* Thousand Oaks, CA: Sage.

Murphy, K. R., Jako, R. A., & Anhalt, R. L. (1993). Nature and consequences of halo error: A critical analysis. *Journal of Applied Psychology, 78*, 218–225.

Myers, J. L., Well, A. D., & Lorch, R. F. (2010). *Research design and statistical analysis* (3rd ed.). New York, NY: Routledge.

Myford, C. M. (2012). Rater cognition research: Some possible directions for the future. *Educational Measurement: Issues and Practice, 31*(3), 48–49.

Myford, C. M., Marr, D. B., & Linacre, J. M. (1996). *Reader calibration and its potential role in equating for the Test of Written English* (TOEFL Research Report No. 95–40). Princeton, NJ: Educational Testing Service.

Myford, C. M., & Wolfe, E. W. (2000). *Strengthening the ties that bind: Improving the linking network in sparsely connected rating designs* (TOEFL Technical Report, TR-15). Princeton, NJ: Educational Testing Service.

Myford, C. M., & Wolfe, E. W. (2002). When raters disagree, then what? Examining a third-rating discrepancy resolution procedure and its utility for identifying unusual patterns of ratings. *Journal of Applied Measurement, 3*, 300–324.

Myford, C. M., & Wolfe, E. W. (2003). Detecting and measuring rater effects using many-facet Rasch measurement: Part I. *Journal of Applied Measurement, 4*, 386–422.

Myford, C. M., & Wolfe, E. W. (2004). Detecting and measuring rater effects using many-facet Rasch measurement: Part II. *Journal of Applied Measurement, 5*, 189–227.

Myford, C. M., & Wolfe, E. W. (2009). Monitoring rater performance over time: A framework for detecting differential accuracy and differential scale category use. *Journal of Educational Measurement, 46*, 371–389.

Newton, P. E., & Shaw, S. D. (2014). *Validity in educational & psychological assessment*. London: Sage.

North, B. (2000). *The development of a common framework scale of language proficiency.* New York, NY: Lang.

North, B. (2008). The CEFR levels and descriptive scales. In L. Taylor & C. J. Weir (Eds.), *Multilingualism and assessment: Achieving transparency, assuring quality, sustaining diversity – Proceedings of the ALTE Berlin Conference May 2005* (pp. 21–66). Cambridge, UK: Cambridge University Press.

North, B., & Jones, N. (2009). *Further material on maintaining standards across languages, contexts and administrations by exploiting teacher judgment and IRT scaling.* Strasbourg, France: Council of Europe/Language Policy Division.

North, B., & Schneider, G. (1998). Scaling descriptors for language proficiency scales. *Language Testing, 15*, 217–262.

Nunnally, J. C. (1978). *Psychometric theory* (2nd ed.). New York, NY: McGraw-Hill.

Ockey, G. J. (2009). The effects of group members' personalities on a test taker's L2 group oral discussion test scores. *Language Testing, 26*, 161–186.

O'Loughlin, K. (2001). *The equivalence of direct and semi-direct speaking tests.* Cambridge, UK: Cambridge University Press.

O'Neill, T. R., & Lunz, M. E. (2000). A method to study rater severity across several administrations. In M. Wilson & G. Engelhard (Eds.), *Objective measurement: Theory into practice* (Vol. 5, pp. 135–146). Stamford, CT: Ablex.

Osterlind, S. J., & Everson, H. T. (2009). *Differential item functioning* (2nd ed.). Los Angeles, CA: Sage.

Ostini, R., & Nering, M. L. (2006). *Polytomous item response theory models.* Thousand Oaks, CA: Sage.

O'Sullivan, B. (2008). *Modelling performance in tests of spoken language.* Frankfurt, Germany: Lang.

O'Sullivan, B., & Rignall, M. (2007). Assessing the value of bias analysis feedback to raters for the IELTS Writing Module. In L. Taylor & P. Falvey (Eds.), *IELTS collected papers: Research in speaking and writing assessment* (pp. 446–478). Cambridge, UK: Cambridge University Press.

Patz, R. J., Junker, B. W., Johnson, M. S., & Mariano, L. T. (2002). The hierarchical rater model for rated test items and its application to large-scale educational assessment data. *Journal of Educational and Behavioral Statistics, 27*, 341–384.

Penfield, R. D. (2014). An NCME instructional module on polytomous item response theory models. *Educational Measurement: Issues and Practice, 33*(1), 36–48.

Penny, J. A., & Johnson, R. L. (2011). The accuracy of performance task scores after resolution of rater disagreement: A Monte Carlo study. *Assessing Writing, 16*, 221–236.

Plake, B. S., & Cizek, G. J. (2012). Variations on a theme: The Modified Angoff, Extended Angoff, and Yes/No standard setting methods. In G. J. Cizek (Ed.), *Setting performance standards: Foundations, methods, and innovations* (2nd ed., pp. 181–199). New York, NY: Routledge.

Purpura, J. E. (2011). Quantitative research methods in assessment and testing. In E. Hinkel (Ed.), *Handbook of research in second language teaching and learning* (Vol. 2, pp. 731–751). New York, NY: Routledge.

R Core Team (2014). R: A language and environment for computing (Version 3.1.2) [Computer software]. Vienna, Austria: R Foundation for Statistical Computing. Retrieved from http://www.R-project.org

Rasch, G. (1980). *Probabilistic models for some intelligence and attainment tests.* Chicago: University of Chicago Press. (Original work published 1960)

Raudenbush, S. W., Bryk, A. S., Cheong, Y. F., Congdon, R., & du Toit, M. (2011). *HLM 7: Hierarchical linear and nonlinear modeling.* Lincolnwood, IL: Scientific Software International.

Reckase, M. D. (2009). *Multidimensional item response theory.* New York, NY: Springer.

Reckase, M. D., Ackerman, T. A., & Carlson, J. E. (1988). Building a unidimensional test using multidimensional items. *Journal of Educational Measurement, 25*, 193–203.

Reed, D. J., & Cohen, A. D. (2001). Revisiting raters and ratings in oral language assessment. In C. Elder et al. (Eds.), *Experimenting with uncertainty: Essays in honour of Alan Davies* (pp. 82–96). Cambridge, UK: Cambridge University Press.

Reise, S. P., Cook, K. F., & Moore, T. M. (2015). Evaluating the impact of multidimensionality on unidimensional item response theory model parameters. In S. P. Reise & D. A. Revicki (Eds.), *Handbook of item response theory modeling: Applications to typical performance assessment* (pp. 13–40). New York, NY: Routledge.

Roberts, C., Rothnie, I., Zoanetti, N., & Crossley, J. (2010). Should candidate scores be adjusted for interviewer stringency or leniency in the multiple mini-interview? *Medical Education, 44*, 690–698.

Roberts, J. K., & Herrington, R. (2007). Demonstration of software programs for estimating multilevel measurement model parameters. In E. V. Smith & R. M. Smith (Eds.), *Rasch measurement: Advanced and specialized applications* (pp. 303–328). Maple Grove, MN: JAM Press.

Robitzsch, A. (2014). Package 'sirt' (Version 1.2) [Computer software and manual]. Retrieved from http://cran.R-project.org/web/packages/sirt/index.html

Rosenbaum, P. R. (1988). Item bundles. *Psychometrika, 53*, 349–359.

Rost, J. (1990). Rasch models in latent classes: An integration of two approaches to item analysis. *Applied Psychological Measurement, 14*, 271–282.

Rost, J. (2001). The growing family of Rasch models. In A. Boomsma, M. A. J. van Duijn, & T. A. B. Snijders (Eds.), *Essays on item response theory* (pp. 25–42). New York, NY: Springer.

Rost, J. (2004). *Lehrbuch Testtheorie, Testkonstruktion* [Textbook test theory, test construction] (2nd ed.). Bern, Switzerland: Huber.

Rost, J., & Carstensen, C. H. (2002). Multidimensional Rasch measurement via item component models and faceted designs. *Applied Psychological Measurement, 26*, 42–56.

Rost, J., & Langeheine, R. (1997). A guide through latent structure models for categorical data. In J. Rost & R. Langeheine (Eds.), *Applications of latent trait and latent class models in the social sciences* (pp. 13–37). Münster, Germany: Waxmann.

Rost, J., & Walter, O. (2006). Multimethod item response theory. In M. Eid & E. Diener (Eds.), *Handbook of multimethod measurement in psychology* (pp. 249–268). Washington, DC: American Psychological Association.

Saal, F. E., Downey, R. G., & Lahey, M. A. (1980). Rating the ratings: Assessing the psychometric quality of rating data. *Psychological Bulletin, 88*, 413–428.

Sasaki, M. (2014). Introspective methods. In A. J. Kunnan (Ed.), *The companion to language assessment: Evaluation, methodology, and interdisciplinary themes* (Vol. 3, pp. 1340–1357). Chichester, UK: Wiley.

Schmidt, K. M., & Embretson, S. E. (2003). Item response theory and measuring abilities. In I. B. Weiner (Series Ed.), J. A. Schinka & W. F. Velicer (Vol. Eds.), *Handbook of psychology: Vol. 2. Research methods in psychology* (pp. 429–445). Hoboken, NJ: Wiley.

Schulz, M. (2002). The standardization of mean-squares. *Rasch Measurement Transactions, 16*, 879.

Schumacker, R. E. (1996, April). *Many-facet Rasch model selection criteria: Examining residuals and more.* Paper presented at the Annual Meeting of the American Educational Research Association, New York, NY. Retrieved from http://eric.ed.gov/?id=ED397117

Schumacker, R. E., & Lunz, M. E. (1997). Interpreting the chi-square statistics reported in the many-faceted Rasch model. *Journal of Outcome Measurement, 1*, 239–257.

Schumacker, R. E., & Smith, E. V. (2007). Reliability: A Rasch perspective. *Educational and Psychological Measurement, 67*, 394–409.

Schuster, C., & Smith, D. A. (2005). Dispersion-weighted kappa: An integrative framework for metric and nominal scale agreement coefficients. *Psychometrika, 70*, 135–146.

Shavelson, R. J., & Webb, N. M. (1991). *Generalizability theory: A primer.* Newbury Park, CA: Sage.

Shaw, S. (2007). Modelling facets of the assessment of Writing within an ESM environment. *Research Notes, 27*, 14–19.

Shohamy, E. (1995). Performance assessment in language testing. *Annual Review of Applied Linguistics, 15*, 188–211.

Shoukri, M. M. (2004). *Measures of interobserver agreement.* Boca Raton, FL: Chapman & Hall/CRC.

Sinharay, S., & Haberman, S. J. (2014). How often is the misfit of item response theory models practically significant? *Educational Measurement: Issues and Practice, 33*(1), 23–35.

Sireci, S. G., Thissen, D., & Wainer, H. (1991). On the reliability of testlet-based tests. *Journal of Educational Measurement, 28*, 237–247.

Smith, A. B., Rush, R., Fallowfield, L. J., Velikova, G., & Sharpe, M. (2008). Rasch fit statistics and sample size considerations for polytomous data. *BMC Medical Research Methodology, 8*(33).

Smith, E. V. (2002). Detecting and evaluating the impact of multidimensionality using item fit statistics and principal component analysis of residuals. *Journal of Applied Measurement, 3*, 205–231.

Smith, E. V. (2004). Metric development and score reporting in Rasch measurement. In E. V. Smith & R. M. Smith (Eds.), *Introduction to Rasch measurement* (pp. 342–365). Maple Grove, MN: JAM Press.

Smith, E. V. (2005). Effect of item redundancy on Rasch item and person estimates. *Journal of Applied Measurement, 6*, 147–163.

Smith, E. V., & Kulikowich, J. M. (2004). An application of generalizability theory and many-facet Rasch measurement using a complex problem-solving skills assessment. *Educational and Psychological Measurement, 64*, 617–639.

Smith, E. V., Wakely, M. B., de Kruif, R. E. L., & Swartz, C. W. (2003). Optimizing rating scales for self-efficacy (and other) research. *Educational and Psychological Measurement, 63*, 369–391.

Smith, R. M. (1991). The distributional properties of Rasch item fit statistics. *Educational and Psychological Measurement, 51*, 541–565.

Smith, R. M. (1996). Polytomous mean-square fit statistics. *Rasch Measurement Transactions, 10*, 516–517.

Smith, R. M. (2004a). Detecting item bias with the Rasch model. *Journal of Applied Measurement, 5*, 430–449.

Smith, R. M. (2004b). Fit analysis in latent trait measurement models. In E. V. Smith & R. M. Smith (Eds.), *Introduction to Rasch measurement* (pp. 73–92). Maple Grove, MN: JAM Press.

Smith, R. M., Schumacker, R. E., & Bush, M. J. (1998). Using item mean squares to evaluate fit to the Rasch model. *Journal of Outcome Measurement, 2*, 66–78.

Spolsky, B. (1995). *Measured words: The development of objective language testing.* Oxford, UK: Oxford University Press.

Stahl, J. A., & Lunz, M. E. (1996). Judge performance reports: Media and message. In G. Engelhard & M. Wilson (Eds.), *Objective measurement: Theory into practice* (Vol. 3, pp. 113–125). Norwood, NJ: Ablex.

Stemler, S. E., & Tsai, J. (2008). Best practices in interrater reliability: Three common approaches. In J. W. Osborne (Ed.), *Best practices in quantitative methods* (pp. 29–49). Los Angeles, CA: Sage.

Stone, G. E. (2006). Whose criterion standard is it anyway? *Journal of Applied Measurement, 7*, 160–169.

Stone, G. E., Beltyukova, S., & Fox, C. M. (2008). Objective standard setting for judge-mediated examinations. *International Journal of Testing, 8*, 180–196.

Su, Y.-H., Sheu, C.-F., & Wang, W.-C. (2007). Computing confidence intervals of item fit statistics in the family of Rasch models using the bootstrap method. *Journal of Applied Measurement, 8*, 190–203.

Sudweeks, R. R., Reeve, S., & Bradshaw, W. S. (2005). A comparison of generalizability theory and many-facet Rasch measurement in an analysis of college sophomore writing. *Assessing Writing, 9*, 239–261.

Suto, I. (2012). A critical review of some qualitative research methods used to explore rater cognition. *Educational Measurement: Issues and Practice, 31*(3), 21–30.

Swaminathan, H., Hambleton, R. K., & Rogers, H. J. (2007). Assessing the fit of item response theory models. In C. R. Rao & S. Sinharay (Eds.), *Psychometrics* (*Handbook of statistics*, Vol. 26, pp. 683–718). Amsterdam: Elsevier.

Sykes, R. C., Ito, K., & Wang, Z. (2008). Effects of assigning raters to items. *Educational Measurement: Issues and Practice, 27*(1), 47–55.

Taube, K. T. (1997). The incorporation of empirical item difficulty data into the Angoff standard-setting procedure. *Evaluation and the Health Professions, 20*, 479–498.

Tennant, A. (2004). Disordered thresholds: An example from the Functional Independence Measure. *Rasch Measurement Transactions, 17*, 945–948.

Tennant, A., & Pallant, J. F. (2006). Unidimensionality matters! (A tale of two Smiths?). *Rasch Measurement Transactions, 20*, 1048–1051.

Thissen, D., Steinberg, L., & Kuang, D. (2002). Quick and easy implementation of the Benjamini–Hochberg procedure for controlling the false positive rate in multiple comparisons. *Journal of Educational and Behavioral Statistics, 27*, 77–83.

Till, H., Ker, J., Myford, C., Stirling, K., & Mires, G. (2015). Constructing and evaluating a validity argument for the final-year ward simulation exercise. *Advances in Health Sciences Education*. Advance online publication. doi: 10.1007/s10459-015-9601-5

Till, H., Myford, C., & Dowell, J. (2013). Improving student selection using multiple mini-interviews with multifaceted Rasch modeling. *Academic Medicine, 88*, 216–223.

Till, H., Myford, C., & Dowell, J. (2015, January). *Building validity arguments for performance assessments used in medical school admission decisions: Investigating examiner performance in the multiple mini-interview process*. Paper presented at the Sixth International Conference on Probabilistic Models for Measurement in Education, Psychology, Social Science and Health, Cape Town, South Africa.

Tinsley, H. E. A., & Weiss, D. J. (1975). Interrater reliability and agreement of subjective judgments. *Journal of Counseling Psychology, 22*, 358–376.

Tinsley, H. E. A., & Weiss, D. J. (2000). Interrater reliability and agreement. In H. E. A. Tinsley & S. D. Brown (Eds.), *Handbook of applied multivariate statistics and mathematical modeling* (pp. 95–124). San Diego, CA: Academic Press.

Turner, C. E. (2014). Mixed methods research. In A. J. Kunnan (Ed.), *The companion to language assessment: Evaluation, methodology, and interdisciplinary themes* (Vol. 3, pp. 1403–1417). Chichester, UK: Wiley.

Van Moere, A. (2006). Validity evidence in a university group oral test. *Language Testing, 23*, 411–440.

Van Moere, A. (2014). Raters and ratings. In A. J. Kunnan (Ed.), *The companion to language assessment: Evaluation, methodology, and interdisciplinary themes* (Vol. 3, pp. 1358–1374). Chichester, UK: Wiley.

Van Nijlen, D., & Janssen, R. (2008). Modeling judgments in the Angoff and contrasting-groups method of standard setting. *Journal of Educational Measurement, 45*, 45–63.

Vaughan, C. (1991). Holistic assessment: What goes on in the rater's mind? In L. Hamp-Lyons (Ed.), *Assessing second language writing in academic contexts* (pp. 111–125). Norwood, NJ: Ablex.

Verheggen, M. M., Muijtjens, A. M. M., Van Os, J., & Schuwirth, L. W. T. (2008). Is an Angoff standard an indication of minimal competence of examinees or of judges? *Advances in Health Sciences Education, 13*, 203–211.

Verhelst, N. D. (2004). Item response theory. In S. Takala (Ed.), *Reference supplement to the preliminary pilot version of the manual for relating language examinations to the Common European Framework of Reference for Languages: Learning, teaching, assessment* (Section G). Strasbourg, France: Council of Europe/Language Policy Division. Retrieved from http://www.coe.int/t/dg4/linguistic/manuel1_EN.asp?#Reference

Verhelst, N. D., & Verstralen, H. H. F. M. (2001). An IRT model for multiple raters. In A. Boomsma, M. A. J. van Duijn, & T. A. B. Snijders (Eds.), *Essays on item response theory* (pp. 89–108). New York, NY: Springer.

Verhelst, N. D., & Verstralen, H. H. F. M. (2008). Some considerations on the partial credit model. *Psicológica, 29*, 229–254.

von Eye, A., & Mun, E. Y. (2005). *Analyzing rater agreement: Manifest variable methods*. Mahwah, NJ: Erlbaum.

Wainer, H., & Kiely, G. L. (1987). Item clusters and computerized adaptive testing: A case for testlets. *Journal of Educational Measurement, 24*, 185–201.

Wang, W.-C. (2000). The simultaneous factorial analysis of differential item functioning. *Methods of Psychological Research Online, 5*, 57–76.

Wang, W.-C., & Chen, C.-T. (2005). Item parameter recovery, standard error estimates, and fit statistics of the WINSTEPS program for the family of Rasch models. *Educational and Psychological Measurement, 65*, 376–404.

Wang, W.-C., & Liu, C.-Y. (2007). Formulation and application of the generalized multilevel facets model. *Educational and Psychological Measurement, 67*, 583–605.

Wang, W.-C., Su, C.-M., & Qiu, X.-L. (2014). Item response models for local dependence among multiple ratings. *Journal of Educational Measurement, 51*, 260–280.

Wang, W.-C., & Wilson, M. (2005a). Exploring local item dependence using a random-effects facet model. *Applied Psychological Measurement, 29*, 296–318.

Wang, W.-C., & Wilson, M. (2005b). The Rasch testlet model. *Applied Psychological Measurement, 29*, 126–149.

Wang, Z., & Yao, L. (2013). *The effects of rater severity and rater distribution on examinees' ability estimation for constructed-response items* (Research Report, RR-13-23). Princeton, NJ: Educational Testing Service.

Weigle, S. C. (1998). Using FACETS to model rater training effects. *Language Testing, 15*, 263–287.

Weigle, S. C. (1999). Investigating rater/prompt interactions in writing assessment: Quantitative and qualitative approaches. *Assessing Writing, 6*, 145–178.

Weigle, S. C. (2002). *Assessing writing.* Cambridge, UK: Cambridge University Press.

Weir, C. J. (2005). *Language testing and validation: An evidence-based approach.* Basingstoke, UK: Palgrave Macmillan.

Wigglesworth, G. (1993). Exploring bias analysis as a tool for improving rater consistency in assessing oral interaction. *Language Testing, 10*, 305–335.

Wigglesworth, G. (2008). Task and performance based assessment. In E. Shohamy & N. H. Hornberger (Eds.), *Encyclopedia of language and education: Vol. 7. Language testing and assessment* (2nd ed., pp. 111–122). New York, NY: Springer.

Wilson, M. (2005). *Constructing measures: An item response modeling approach.* Mahwah, NJ: Erlbaum.

Wilson, M. (2011). Some notes on the term: "Wright map". *Rasch Measurement Transactions, 25*, 1331.

Wilson, M., & Adams, R. J. (1995). Rasch models for item bundles. *Psychometrika, 60*, 181–198.

Wilson, M., & Case, H. (2000). An examination of variation in rater severity over time: A study in rater drift. In M. Wilson & G. Engelhard (Eds.), *Objective measurement: Theory into practice* (pp. 113–133). Stamford, CT: Ablex.

Wilson, M., & Hoskens, M. (2001). The rater bundle model. *Journal of Educational and Behavioral Statistics, 26*, 283–306.

Wimsatt, W. C. (2007). *Re-engineering philosophy for limited beings: Piecewise approximations to reality.* Cambridge, MA: Harvard University Press.

Wind, S. A., & Engelhard, G. (2013). How invariant and accurate are domain ratings in writing assessment? *Assessing Writing, 18*, 278–299.

Winke, P., Gass, S., & Myford, C. (2011). *The relationship between raters' prior language study and the evaluation of foreign language speech samples* (TOEFL iBT Research Report, RR-11-30). Princeton, NJ: Educational Testing Service.

Winke, P., Gass, S., & Myford, C. (2013). Raters' L2 background as a potential source of bias in rating oral performance. *Language Testing, 30*, 231–252.

Wolfe, E. W. (1997). The relationship between essay reading style and scoring proficiency in a psychometric scoring system. *Assessing Writing, 4*, 83–106.

Wolfe, E. W. (2000). Equating and item banking with the Rasch model. *Journal of Applied Measurement, 1*, 409–434.

Wolfe, E. W. (2004). Identifying rater effects using latent trait models. *Psychology Science, 46*, 35–51.

Wolfe, E. W. (2008). RBF.sas (Rasch Bootstrap Fit): A SAS macro for estimating critical values for Rasch model fit statistics. *Applied Psychological Measurement, 32*, 585–586.

Wolfe, E. W. (2009). Item and rater analysis of constructed response items via the multi-faceted Rasch model. *Journal of Applied Measurement, 10*, 335–347.

Wolfe, E. W. (2013). A bootstrap approach to evaluating person and item fit to the Rasch model. *Journal of Applied Measurement, 14*, 1–9.

Wolfe, E. W., Chiu, C. W. T., & Myford, C. M. (2000). Detecting rater effects in simulated data with a multifaceted Rasch rating scale model. In M. Wilson & G. Engelhard (Eds.), *Objective measurement: Theory into practice* (Vol. 5, pp. 147–164). Stamford, CT: Ablex.

Wolfe, E. W., & Dobria, L. (2008). Applications of the multifaceted Rasch model. In J. W. Osborne (Ed.), *Best practices in quantitative methods* (pp. 71–85). Los Angeles, CA: Sage.

Wolfe, E. W., & McVay, A. (2012). Application of latent trait models to identifying substantively interesting raters. *Educational Measurement: Issues and Practice, 31*(3), 31–37.

Wolfe, E. W., Moulder, B. C., & Myford, C. M. (2001). Detecting differential rater functioning over time (DRIFT) using a Rasch multi-faceted rating scale model. *Journal of Applied Measurement, 2*, 256–280.

Wolfe, E. W., Myford, C. M., Engelhard, G., & Manalo, J. R. (2007). *Monitoring reader performance and DRIFT in the AP English Literature and Composition examination using benchmark essays* (College Board Research Report No. 2007-2). New York, NY: College Board.

Wolfe, E. W., & Smith, E. V. (2007a). Instrument development tools and activities for measure validation using Rasch models: Part I – Instrument development tools. In E. V. Smith & R. M. Smith (Eds.), *Rasch measurement: Advanced and specialized applications* (pp. 202–242). Maple Grove, MN: JAM Press.

Wolfe, E. W., & Smith, E. V. (2007b). Instrument development tools and activities for measure validation using Rasch models: Part II – Validation activities. In E. V. Smith & R. M. Smith (Eds.), *Rasch measurement: Advanced and specialized applications* (pp. 243–290). Maple Grove, MN: JAM Press.

Wolfe, E. W., & Song, T. (2014). Rater effect comparability in local independence and rater bundle models. *Journal of Applied Measurement, 15*, 152–159.

Wolfe, F., Macintosh, R., Kreiner, S., Lange, R., Graves, R., & Linacre, J. M. (2006). Multiple significance tests. *Rasch Measurement Transactions, 19*, 1044.

Woods, A., & Baker, R. (1985). Item response theory. *Language Testing, 2*, 117–140.

Wright, B. D. (1967, October). *Sample-free test calibration and person measurement.* Paper presented at the ETS Invitational Conference on Testing Problems, Princeton, NJ. Retrieved from http://www.rasch.org/memo1.htm

Wright, B. D. (1995). Which standard error? *Rasch Measurement Transactions, 9*, 436.

Wright, B. D. (1996). Reliability and separation. *Rasch Measurement Transactions, 9*, 472.

Wright, B. D. (1999). Fundamental measurement for psychology. In S. E. Embretson & S. L. Hershberger (Eds.), *The new rules of measurement: What every psychologist and educator should know* (pp. 65–104). Mahwah, NJ: Erlbaum.

Wright, B. D., & Andrich, D. A. (1987). Rasch and Wright: The early years. *Rasch Measurement Transactions, Pre-History*, 1–4.

Wright, B. D., & Linacre, J. M. (1994). Reasonable mean-square fit values. *Rasch Measurement Transactions, 8*, 370.

Wright, B. D., & Masters, G. N. (1982). *Rating scale analysis.* Chicago: MESA Press.

Wright, B. D., & Masters, G. N. (2002). Number of person or item strata. *Rasch Measurement Transactions, 16*, 888.

Wright, B. D., & Mok, M. M. C. (2004). An overview of the family of Rasch measurement models. In E. V. Smith & R. M. Smith (Eds.), *Introduction to Rasch measurement* (pp. 1–24). Maple Grove, MN: JAM Press.

Wright, B. D., & Panchapakesan, N. (1969). A procedure for sample-free item analysis. *Educational and Psychological Measurement, 29*, 23–48.

Wright, B. D., & Stone, M. H. (1979). *Best test design.* Chicago: MESA Press.

Wu, M., & Adams, R. J. (2013). Properties of Rasch residual fit statistics. *Journal of Applied Measurement, 14*, 339–355.

Xi, X. (2010). How do we go about investigating test fairness? *Language Testing, 27*, 147–170.

Yan, X. (2014). An examination of rater performance on a local oral English proficiency test: A mixed-methods approach. *Language Testing, 31*, 501–527.

Yen, W. M., & Fitzpatrick, A. R. (2006). Item response theory. In R. L. Brennan (Ed.), *Educational measurement* (4th ed., pp. 111–153). Westport, CT: American Council on Education/Praeger.

Zegers, F. E. (1991). Coefficients for interrater agreement. *Applied Psychological Measurement, 15*, 321–333.

Zhu, W. (2002). A confirmatory study of Rasch-based optimal categorization of a rating scale. *Journal of Applied Measurement, 3*, 1–15.

Zhu, W., Updyke, W. F., & Lewandowski, C. (1997). Post-hoc Rasch analysis of optimal categorization of an ordered-response scale. *Journal of Outcome Measurement, 1*, 286–304.

Author Index

T

U

V

W

Subject Index

S

Language Testing and Evaluation

Series editors: Rüdiger Grotjahn and Günther Sigott

Vol. 1 Günther Sigott: Towards Identifying the C-Test Construct. 2004.

Vol. 2 Carsten Röver. Testing ESL Pragmatics. Development and Validation of a Web-Based Assessment Battery. 2005.

Vol. 3 Tom Lumley: Assessing Second Language Writing. The Rater's Perspective. 2005.

Vol. 4 Annie Brown: Interviewer Variability in Oral Proficiency Interviews. 2005.

Vol. 5 Jianda Liu: Measuring Interlanguage Pragmatic Knowledge of EFL Learners. 2006.

Vol. 6 Rüdiger Grotjahn (Hrsg. / ed.): Der C-Test: Theorie, Empirie, Anwendungen/The C-Test: Theory, Empirical Research, Applications. 2006.

Vol. 7 Vivien Berry: Personality Differences and Oral Test Performance. 2007.

Vol. 8 John O'Dwyer: Formative Evaluation for Organisational Learning. A Case Study of the Management of a Process of Curriculum Development. 2008.

Vol. 9 Aek Phakiti: Strategic Competence and EFL Reading Test Performance. A Structural Equation Modeling Approach. 2007.

Vol. 10 Gábor Szabó: Applying Item Response Theory in Language Test Item Bank Building. 2008.

Vol. 11 John M. Norris: Validity Evaluation in Language Assessment. 2008.

Vol. 12 Barry O'Sullivan: Modelling Performance in Tests of Spoken Language. 2008.

Vol. 13 Annie Brown / Kathryn Hill (eds.): Tasks and Criteria in Performance Assessment. Proceedings of the 28th Language Testing Research Colloquium. 2009.

Vol. 14 Ildikó Csépes: Measuring Oral Proficiency through Paired-Task Performance. 2009.

Vol. 15 Dina Tsagari: The Complexity of Test Washback. An Empirical Study. 2009.

Vol. 16 Spiros Papageorgiou: Setting Performance Standards in Europe. The Judges' Contribution to Relating Language Examinations to the Common European Framework of Reference. 2009.

Vol. 17 Ute Knoch: Diagnostic Writing Assessment. The Development and Validation of a Rating Scale. 2009.

Vol. 18 Rüdiger Grotjahn (Hrsg. / ed.): Der C-Test: Beiträge aus der aktuellen Forschung/The C-Test: Contributions from Current Research. 2010.

Vol. 19 Fred Dervin / Eija Suomela-Salmi (eds. / éds): New Approaches to Assessing Language and (Inter-)Cultural Competences in Higher Education / Nouvelles approches de l'évaluation des compétences langagières et (inter-)culturelles dans l'enseignement supérieur. 2010.

Vol. 20 Ana Maria Ducasse: Interaction in Paired Oral Proficiency Assessment in Spanish. Rater and Candidate Input into Evidence Based Scale Development and Construct Definition. 2010.

Vol. 21 Luke Harding: Accent and Listening Assessment. A Validation Study of the Use of Speakers with L2 Accents on an Academic English Listening Test. 2011.

Vol. 22 Thomas Eckes: Introduction to Many-Facet Rasch Measurement. Analyzing and Evaluating Rater-Mediated Assessments. 2011. 2nd Revised and Updated Edition. 2015.

Vol. 23 Gabriele Kecker: Validierung von Sprachprüfungen. Die Zuordnung des TestDaF zum Gemeinsamen europäischen Referenzrahmen für Sprachen. 2011.

Vol. 24 Lyn May: Interaction in a Paired Speaking Test. The Rater´s Perspective. 2011.

Vol. 25 Dina Tsagari / Ildikó Csépes (eds.): Classroom-Based Language Assessment. 2011.

Vol. 26 Dina Tsagari / Ildikó Csépes (eds.): Collaboration in Language Testing and Assessment. 2012.

Vol. 27 Kathryn Hill: Classroom-Based Assessment in the School Foreign Language Classroom. 2012.

Vol. 28 Dina Tsagari / Salomi Papadima-Sophocleous / Sophie Ioannou-Georgiou (eds.): International Experiences in Language Testing and Assessment. Selected Papers in Memory of Pavlos Pavlou. 2013.

Vol. 29 Dina Tsagari / Roelof van Deemter (eds.): Assessment Issues in Language Translation and Interpreting. 2013.

Vol. 30 Fumiyo Nakatsuhara: The Co-construction of Conversation in Group Oral Tests. 2013.

Vol. 31 Veronika Timpe: Assessing Intercultural Language Learning. The Dependence of Receptive Sociopragmatic Competence and Discourse Competence on Learning Opportunities and Input. 2013.

Vol. 32 Florian Kağan Meyer: Language Proficiency Testing for Chinese as a Foreign Language. An Argument-Based Approach for Validating the Hanyu Shuiping Kaoshi (HSK). 2014.

Vol. 33 Katrin Wisniewski: Die Validität der Skalen des Gemeinsamen europäischen Referenzrahmens für Sprachen. Eine empirische Untersuchung der Flüssigkeits- und Wortschatzskalen des GeRS am Beispiel des Italienischen und des Deutschen. 2014.

Vol. 34 Rüdiger Grotjahn (Hrsg./ed.): Der C-Test: Aktuelle Tendenzen/The C-Test: Current Trends. 2014.

Vol. 35 Carsten Roever / Catriona Fraser / Catherine Elder: Testing ESL Sociopragmatics. Development and Validation of a Web-based Test Battery. 2014.

Vol. 36 Trisevgeni Liontou: Computational Text Analysis and Reading Comprehension Exam Complexity. Towards Automatic Text Classification. 2015.

www.peterlang.com

Lightning Source UK Ltd.
Milton Keynes UK
UKHW012148051222
413422UK00005B/71

9 783631 656150